Neonatal Hyperbilirubinemia in Preterm Neonates

Editors

DAVID K. STEVENSON
VINOD K. BHUTANI

CLINICS IN PERINATOLOGY

www.perinatology.theclinics.com

Consulting Editor
LUCKY JAIN

June 2016 • Volume 43 • Number 2

ELSEVIER

1600 John F. Kennedy Boulevard • Suite 1800 • Philadelphia, Pennsylvania, 19103-2899

http://www.theclinics.com

CLINICS IN PERINATOLOGY Volume 43, Number 2
June 2016 ISSN 0095-5108, ISBN-13: 978-0-323-44628-0

Editor: Kerry Holland
Developmental Editor: Casey Jackson

Clinics in Perinatology (ISSN 0095-5108) is published quarterly by Elsevier Inc., 360 Park Avenue South, New York, NY 10010-1710. Months of issue are March, June, September, and December. Business and Editorial Offices: 1600 John F. Kennedy Blvd., Ste. 1800, Philadelphia, PA 19103-2899. Customer Service Office: 3251 Riverport Lane, Maryland Heights, MO 63043. Periodicals postage paid at New York, NY and additional mailing offices. Subscription prices are $290.00 per year (US individuals), $502.00 per year (US institutions), $340.00 per year (Canadian individuals), $614.00 per year (Canadian institutions), $420.00 per year (international individuals), $614.00 per year (international institutions), $100.00 per year (US students), and $195.00 per year (Canadian and international students). International air speed delivery is included in all Clinics subscription prices. All prices are subject to change without notice. **POSTMASTER:** Send address changes to *Clinics in Perinatology*, Elsevier Health Sciences Division, Subscription Customer Service, 3251 Riverport Lane, Maryland Heights, MO 63043. **Customer Service: Telephone: 1-800-654-2452** (U.S. and Canada); **1-314-447-8871** (outside U.S. and Canada). **Fax: 1-314-447-8029. E-mail: journalscustomerservice-usa@elsevier.com** (for print support); **journalsonlinesupport-usa@elsevier.com** (for online support).

Reprints. For copies of 100 or more, of articles in this publication, please contact the Commercial Reprints Department, Elsevier Inc., 360 Park Avenue South, New York, NY 10010-1710. Tel. 212-633-3874; Fax: 212-633-3820; E-mail: reprints@elsevier.com.

Clinics in Perinatology is also pubilshed in Spanish by McGraw-Hill Interamericana Editores S.A., P.O. Box 5-237, 06500 Mexico D.F., Mexico.

Clinics in Perinatology is covered in *MEDLINE/PubMed (Index Medicus) Current Contents, Excepta Medica, BIOSIS and ISI/BIOMED.*

Contributors

CONSULTING EDITOR

LUCKY JAIN, MD, MBA
Richard W. Blumberg Professor and Interim Chair, Emory University School of Medicine, Department of Pediatrics, Executive Medical Director and Interim Chief Academic Officer, Children's Healthcare of Atlanta, Atlanta, Georgia

EDITORS

DAVID K. STEVENSON, MD
Harold K. Faber Professor of Pediatrics, Senior Associate Dean for Maternal and Child Health, Stanford University School of Medicine, Department of Pediatrics, Division of Neonatal and Developmental Medicine, Stanford, California

VINOD K. BHUTANI, MD
Professor of Pediatrics, Division of Neonatal and Developmental Medicine, Department of Pediatrics, Stanford Children's Health, Lucile Packard Children's Hospital, Stanford University School of Medicine, Stanford, California

AUTHORS

SANJIV B. AMIN, MBBS, MD, MS
Associate Professor, Department of Pediatrics, Division of Neonatology, University of Rochester School of Medicine and Dentistry, Rochester, New York

YASSAR H. ARAIN, MD
Neonatal-Perinatal Medicine Fellow, Division of Neonatal and Developmental Medicine, Department of Pediatrics, Stanford University School of Medicine, Stanford, California

CODY C. ARNOLD, MD, MSc, MPH
Associate Professor, Department of Pediatrics, University of Texas Health Science Center at Houston, Houston, Texas

VINOD K. BHUTANI, MD
Professor of Pediatrics, Division of Neonatal and Developmental Medicine, Department of Pediatrics, Stanford Children's Health, Lucile Packard Children's Hospital, Stanford University School of Medicine, Stanford, California

ROBERT D. CHRISTENSEN, MD
Division of Hematology/Oncology, Department of Pediatrics, Primary Children's Hospital; Women and Newborn's Clinical Program, Division of Neonatology, Department of Pediatrics, Intermountain Healthcare, University of Utah School of Medicine, Salt Lake City, Utah

ANNA D. CUNNINGHAM, BS
Department of Chemical and Systems Biology, Stanford University, Stanford, California

GLENN GOURLEY, MD
Professor, Pediatric Gastroenterology, Department of Pediatrics, University of Minnesota, Minneapolis, Minnesota

CATHY HAMMERMAN, MD
Faculty of Medicine, The Hebrew University of Jerusalem; Department of Neonatology, Shaare Zedek Medical Center, Jerusalem, Israel

THOR WILLY RUUD HANSEN, MD, PhD, MHA, FAAP
Faculty of Medicine, Division of Paediatric and Adolescent Medicine, Oslo University Hospital, Institute of Clinical Medicine, University of Oslo, Oslo, Norway

SUNHEE HWANG, PhD
Department of Chemical and Systems Biology, Stanford University, Stanford, California

MICHAEL KAPLAN, MB ChB
Faculty of Medicine, The Hebrew University of Jerusalem; Department of Neonatology, Shaare Zedek Medical Center, Jerusalem, Israel

ANGELO A. LAMOLA, PhD
Consulting Professor, Division of Neonatal and Developmental Medicine, Department of Pediatrics, Stanford University School of Medicine, Stanford, California

DARIA MOCHLY-ROSEN, PhD
Department of Chemical and Systems Biology, Stanford University, Stanford, California

JOHN S. OGHALAI, MD
Department of Otolaryngology – Head and Neck Surgery, Stanford University, Stanford, California

CRISTEN OLDS, MD
Department of Otolaryngology – Head and Neck Surgery, Stanford University, Stanford, California

JONATHAN P. PALMA, MD, MS
Clinical Assistant Professor, Division of Neonatal and Developmental Medicine, Department of Pediatrics, Stanford University School of Medicine, Stanford, California; Department of Clinical Informatics, Stanford Children's Health, Palo Alto, California

CLAUDIA PEDROZA, PhD
Assistant Professor, Department of Pediatrics, University of Texas Health Science Center at Houston, Houston, Texas

KATIE SATROM, MD
Fellow, Division of Neonatology, Department of Pediatrics, University of Minnesota, Minneapolis, Minnesota

DAVID K. STEVENSON, MD
Harold K. Faber Professor of Pediatrics, Senior Associate Dean for Maternal and Child Health, Stanford University School of Medicine, Department of Pediatrics, Division of Neonatal and Developmental Medicine, Stanford, California

JON E. TYSON, MD, MPH
Professor, Department of Pediatrics, University of Texas Health Science Center at Houston, Houston, Texas

JON F. WATCHKO, MD
Professor of Pediatrics, Obstetrics, Gynecology and Reproductive Sciences, Division of Newborn Medicine, Department of Pediatrics, Magee-Womens Hospital, Children's Hospital of Pittsburgh, Magee-Womens Research Institute, University of Pittsburgh School of Medicine, Pittsburgh, Pennsylvania

RONALD J. WONG, BS
Senior Research Scientist, Division of Neonatal and Developmental Medicine, Department of Pediatrics, Stanford Children's Health, Lucile Packard Children's Hospital, Stanford University School of Medicine, Stanford, California

HASSAN M. YAISH, MD
Division of Hematology/Oncology, Department of Pediatrics, Primary Children's Hospital, University of Utah School of Medicine, Salt Lake City, Utah

Contents

> Preterm neonates with increased bilirubin production loads are more likely to sustain adverse outcomes due to either neurotoxicity or overtreatment with phototherapy and/or exchange transfusion. Clinicians should rely on expert consensus opinions to guide timely and effective interventions until there is better evidence to refine bilirubin-induced neurologic dysfunction or benefits of bilirubin. In this article, we review the evolving evidence for bilirubin-induced brain injury in preterm infants and highlight the clinical approaches that minimize the risk of bilirubin neurotoxicity.

> Hemolysis can be an important cause of hyperbilirubinemia in premature and term neonates. It can result from genetic abnormalities intrinsic to or factors exogenous to normal to red blood cells (RBCs). Hemolysis can lead to a relatively rapid increase in total serum/plasma bilirubin, hyperbilirubinemia that is somewhat slow to fall with phototherapy, or hyperbilirubinemia that is likely to rebound after phototherapy. Laboratory methods for diagnosing hemolysis are more difficult to apply, or less conclusive, in preterm infants. Transfusion of donor RBCs can present a bilirubin load that must be metabolized. Genetic causes can be identified by next-generation sequencing panels.

> Total serum/plasma bilirubin (TB), the biochemical measure currently used to evaluate and manage hyperbilirubinemia, is not a useful predictor of bilirubin-induced neurotoxicity in premature infants. Altered bilirubin–albumin binding in premature infants limits the usefulness of TB in premature infants. In this article, bilirubin–albumin binding, a modifying factor for bilirubin-induced neurotoxicity, in premature infants is reviewed.

in preterm neonates, and although multifactorial in nature, is often associated with marked hypoalbuminemia.

Although hyperbilirubinemia is extremely common among neonates and is usually mild and transient, it sometimes leads to bilirubin-induced neurologic damage (BIND). The auditory pathway is highly sensitive to the effects of elevated total serum/plasma bilirubin (TB) levels, with damage manifesting clinically as auditory neuropathy spectrum disorder. Compared to full-term neonates, preterm neonates are more susceptible to BIND and suffer adverse effects at lower TB levels with worse long-term outcomes. Furthermore, although standardized guidelines for management of hyperbilirubinemia exist for term and late preterm neonates, similar guidelines for neonates less than 35 weeks gestational age are limited.

Prematurity and glucose-6-phosphate dehydrogenase (G6PD) deficiency are risk factors for neonatal hyperbilirubinemia. The 2 conditions may interact additively or synergistically, contributing to extreme hyperbilirubinemia, with the potential for bilirubin neurotoxicity. This hyperbilirubinemia is the result of sudden, unpredictable, and acute episodes of hemolysis in combination with immaturity of bilirubin elimination, primarily of conjugation. Avoidance of contact with known triggers of hemolysis in G6PD-deficient individuals will prevent some, but not all, episodes of hemolysis. All preterm infants with G6PD deficiency should be vigilantly observed for the development of jaundice both in hospital and after discharge home.

Hyperbilirubinemia occurs frequently in newborns, and in severe cases can progress to kernicterus and permanent developmental disorders. Glucose-6-phosphate dehydrogenase (G6PD) deficiency, one of the most common human enzymopathies, is a major risk factor for hyperbilirubinemia and greatly increases the risk of kernicterus even in the developed world. Therefore, a novel treatment for kernicterus is needed, especially for G6PD-deficient newborns. Oxidative stress is a hallmark of bilirubin toxicity in the brain. We propose that the activation of G6PD via a small molecule chaperone is a potential strategy to increase endogenous defense against bilirubin-induced oxidative stress and prevent kernicterus.

Cholestasis in preterm infants has a multifactorial etiology. Risk factors include degree of prematurity, lack of enteral feeding, intestinal injury,

prolonged use of parenteral nutrition (PN), and sepsis. Soy-based parenteral lipid emulsions have been implicated in the pathophysiology of
PN-associated liver injury. Inflammation plays an important role. Medical
therapies are used; however, their effects have not consistently proven
effective. Evaluation of cholestasis involves laboratory work; direct bilirubin levels are used for diagnosis and trending. Adverse outcomes
include risk for hepatobiliary dysfunction, irreversible liver failure, and
death. Early enteral feedings as tolerated is the best way to prevent and
manage cholestasis.

Premie BiliRecs is a novel electronic clinical decision support tool for the
management of hyperbilirubinemia in moderately preterm infants less
than 35 weeks gestational age. It serves to operationalize and automate
current expert consensus-based guidelines, and to aid in the generation
of new practice-based evidence to inform future guidelines.

PROGRAM OBJECTIVE

The goal of *Clinics in Perinatology* is to keep practicing perinatologists, neonatologists, obstetricians, practicing physicians and residents up to date with current clinical practice in perinatology by providing timely articles reviewing the state of the art in patient care.

TARGET AUDIENCE

Perinatologists, neonatologists, obstetricians, practicing physicians, residents and healthcare professionals who provide patient care utilizing findings from *Clinics in Perinatology.*

LEARNING OBJECTIVES

Upon completion of this activity, participants will be able to:
1. Review management strategies for hyperbilirubinemia in infants.
2. Discuss the use of phototherapy in neonates with hyperbilirubinemia.
3. Recognize complications of hyperbilirubinemia.

ACCREDITATION

The Elsevier Office of Continuing Medical Education (EOCME) is accredited by the Accreditation Council for Continuing Medical Education (ACCME) to provide continuing medical education for physicians.

The EOCME designates this enduring material for a maximum of 15 *AMA PRA Category 1 Credit*(s)™. Physicians should claim only the credit commensurate with the extent of their participation in the activity.

All other health care professionals requesting continuing education credit for this enduring material will be issued a certificate of participation.

DISCLOSURE OF CONFLICTS OF INTEREST

The EOCME assesses conflict of interest with its instructors, faculty, planners, and other individuals who are in a position to control the content of CME activities. All relevant conflicts of interest that are identified are thoroughly vetted by EOCME for fair balance, scientific objectivity, and patient care recommendations. EOCME is committed to providing its learners with CME activities that promote improvements or quality in healthcare and not a specific proprietary business or a commercial interest.

The planning committee, staff, authors and editors listed below have identified no financial relationships or relationships to products or devices they or their spouse/life partner have with commercial interest related to the content of this CME activity:
Sanjiv B. Amin, MBBS, MD, MS; Yassar H. Arain, MD; Cody C. Arnold, MD, MSc, MPH; Vinod K. Bhutani, MD; Robert D. Christensen, MD; Anna D. Cunningham, BS; Anjali Fortna; Glenn Gourley, MD; Cathy Hammerman, MD; Thor Willy Ruud Hansen, MD, PhD, MHA, FAAP; Kerry Holland; Sunhee Hwang, PhD; Lucky Jain, MD, MBA; Michael Kaplan, MB ChB; Angelo A. Lamola, PhD; Daria Mochly-Rosen, PhD; Palani Murugesan; John S. Oghalai, MD; Cristen Olds, MD; Jonathan P. Palma, MD, MS; Claudia Pedroza, PhD; Katie Satrom, MD; David K. Stevenson, MD; Megan Suermann; Jon E. Tyson, MD, MPH; Jon F. Watchko, MD; Ronald J. Wong, BS; Hassan M. Yaish, MD.

UNAPPROVED/OFF-LABEL USE DISCLOSURE

The EOCME requires CME faculty to disclose to the participants:
1. When products or procedures being discussed are off-label, unlabelled, experimental, and/or investigational (not US Food and Drug Administration [FDA] approved); and
2. Any limitations on the information presented, such as data that are preliminary or that represent ongoing research, interim analyses, and/or unsupported opinions. Faculty may discuss information about pharmaceutical agents that is outside of FDA-approved labelling. This information is intended solely for CME and is not intended to promote off-label use of these medications. If you have any questions, contact the medical affairs department of the manufacturer for the most recent prescribing information.

TO ENROLL

To enroll in the *Clinics in Perinatology* Continuing Medical Education program, call customer service at 1-800-654-2452 or sign up online at http://www.theclinics.com/home/cme. The CME program is available to subscribers for an additional annual fee of $235 USD.

METHOD OF PARTICIPATION

In order to claim credit, participants must complete the following:
1. Complete enrolment as indicated above.

2. Read the activity.
3. Complete the CME Test and Evaluation. Participants must achieve a score of 70% on the test. All CME Tests and Evaluations must be completed online.

CME INQUIRIES/SPECIAL NEEDS

For all CME inquiries or special needs, please contact elsevierCME@elsevier.com.

CLINICS IN PERINATOLOGY

Foreword

Why the Premature Brain Is More Prone to Bilirubin-induced Injury

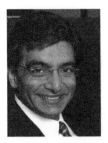

Lucky Jain, MD, MBA
Consulting Editor

For premature babies, the initial start in life can be tough! Just as they are recovering from respiratory distress and cardiovascular issues, a new problem looms large: hyperbilirubinemia! And to make matters worse, it turns out that bilirubin-induced brain damage may be more common than originally thought, and that thresholds for toxicity vary widely even among preterm infants of similar gestational age.[1] Indeed, the presence of comorbid conditions increases the propensity for injury, as does the loss of albumin and/or its bilirubin-binding capacity.[2] Given how many of these factors commonly interplay in the sickest of our preterm infants, it is hard to imagine how any of them escape injury.

Because chronic bilirubin encephalopathy–associated brain injury can be irreversible (**Fig. 1**),[3] clinicians and scientists have directed their attention toward primary prevention of the disorder. However, factors leading to moderate or severe hyperbilirubinemia in preterm infants differ from those in term infants. Higher red blood cell turnover and reduced bilirubin conjugation are understandable, but attention has been directed to reduced bilirubin binding capacity and factors that make the blood-brain barrier more permeable to bilirubin passage.[4] There is need for better understanding of what makes the endothelial junctions more leaky and the role of pericyte dysfunction.[5] This could provide interventions that stabilize the barrier even in the face of persistent hyperbilirubinemia. Early identification of bilirubin-induced neurologic dysfunction is also critical if we are to succeed in preventing ongoing injury. This is particularly true in low-bilirubin kernicterus, where injury is often totally unexpected.[6]

In this issue of *Clinics in Perinatology*, Drs Bhutani and Stevenson have put a together a state-of-the-art compilation of articles related to hyperbilirubinemia in the preterm infant. The articles tackle tough issues discussed above and offer a single source of complete information on this topic. Where evidence-based guidelines are

Clin Perinatol 43 (2016) xv–xvi
http://dx.doi.org/10.1016/j.clp.2016.03.002
0095-5108/16/$ – see front matter © 2016 Published by Elsevier Inc.

perinatology.theclinics.com

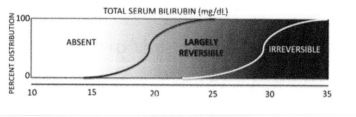

Neurotoxicity Risk Factors:	IMPAIRED CELL FUNCTION:		
•Hemolytic Disease	POSSIBLE RISK OF BIND BASED	RISK OF CELL	CELL DEATH
•G6PD Deficiency	NEONATAL VULNERABILITIES:	DEATH	LIKELY
•Asphyxia	GA, BBC AND OTHERS		
•Significant Lethargy			
•Temperature Instability			
•Sepsis, Acidosis	RISK OF BILIRUBIN NEUROTOXICITY		
•Albumin <3.0 g/dL			

Fig. 1. Model for reversible bilirubin neurotoxicity. BBC, bilirubin binding capacity; GA, gestational age; G6P, glucose-6-phosphate dehydrogenase. (*Reprinted from* Bhutani VK, Johnson-Hamerman L. The clinical syndrome of bilirubin-induced neurologic dysfunction. Semin Fetal Neonatal Med 2015;20:7; with permission.)

not available, the editors have brought in some of the best-known experts in this field to drive consensus-based recommendations.

I also want to thank the editors, authors, and the publishing team at Elsevier (Kerry Holland and Casey Jackson) for bringing together yet another superb issue of the *Clinics in Perinatology* for you.

Lucky Jain, MD, MBA
Emory University School of Medicine
Department of Pediatrics
Children's Healthcare of Atlanta
2015 Uppergate Drive
Atlanta, GA 30322, USA

E-mail address:
ljain@emory.edu

REFERENCES

1. Wusthoff CJ, Loe IM. Impact of bilirubin-induced neurologic dysfunction on neurodevelopmental outcomes. Semin Fetal Neonatal Med 2015;20:52–7.
2. Maisels MJ, Watchko JF, Bhutani VK, et al. An approach to the management of hyperbilirubinemia in the preterm infant less than 35 weeks gestation. J Perinatol 2012;32:660–4.
3. Bhutani VK, Johnson-Hamerman L. The clinical syndrome of bilirubin-induced neurologic dysfunction. Semin Fetal Neonatal Med 2015;20:6–13.
4. Brito MA, Palmela I, Cardoso FL, et al. Blood-brain barrier and bilirubin: clinical aspects and experimental data. Arch Med Res 2014;45:660–76.
5. Brites D, Fernandes A. Bilirubin induced neural impairment: a special focus on myelination, age related windows of susceptibility and associated co-morbidities. Semin Fetal Neonatal Med 2015;20:14–9.
6. Watchko JF, Maisels MJ. The enigma of low bilirubin kernicterus in premature infants: why does it still occur, and is it preventable? Semin Perinatol 2014;38:397–406.

Preface

Preterm Neonates: Beyond the Guidelines for Neonatal Hyperbilirubinemia

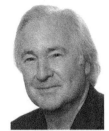 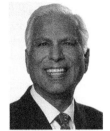

David K. Stevenson, MD   Vinod K. Bhutani, MD
Editors

The management of neonatal hyperbilirubinemia in late preterm neonates between 35 and 37 weeks gestation is addressed by the American Academy of Pediatrics (AAP) 2004 guideline for "Management of hyperbilirubinemia in the newborn infant 35 or more weeks of gestation."[1,2] The extension of the AAP guideline to late preterm infants stretches the limits of the evidence supporting how best to manage these jaundiced infants, but it nonetheless presents a consensus of experts who have taken into account what is known about neonatal hyperbilirubinemia and combined it with their experience and good sense. This issue of *Clinics in Perinatology* ventures further into this uncertain territory of neonatology and reflects a collection of expert opinions about the risks of hyperbilirubinemia facing all preterm infants, and especially those less than 35 weeks gestation. For example, preterm infants are known to have a shorter red blood cell lifespan and a greater transient impairment of bilirubin conjugation, which is necessary for excretion of bilirubin. Due to the former, preterm infants already have some degree of hemolysis, putting them at an increased risk for developing extremely high bilirubin levels for a protracted period beyond the first several days of life. Thus, other causes of hemolysis in preterm infants represent an especially dangerous circumstance with the potential to exceed rapidly the bilirubin binding capacity (BBC), which is also reduced. The preterm infant is also much more likely to be metabolically unstable in the early transition after birth, further jeopardizing binding affinity, which is known to be temporarily impaired as well. The articles addressing neonatal hemolysis and BBC provide insight into these developmental limitations. Phototherapy remains the mainstay for treating hyperbilirubinemia in preterm neonates. Several articles focus on phototherapy and suggest new approaches to phototherapy in preterm infants that may be not only safer, but also more effective. Deafness is a major morbidity among preterm infants and probably has many causes.

Clin Perinatol 43 (2016) xvii–xviii
http://dx.doi.org/10.1016/j.clp.2016.01.013
0095-5108/16/$ – see front matter © 2016 Published by Elsevier Inc.

perinatology.theclinics.com

Neonatal hyperbilirubinemia, however, is discussed as one of the most significant contributing causes, and it is apparent that preterm infants are more susceptible to such injury. The identification of auditory dysfunction may be important in deciding when to treat hyperbilirubinemia as well as when treatment is effective. Nonetheless, it is often difficult to identify bilirubin-induced neurologic dysfunction (BIND) in a preterm infant whose developmental state may restrict the identification of neurologic findings that the clinician encounters, so that the classic kernicterus syndrome, nonspecific as it is in any case, may not be recognized easily. Glucose-6-phosphate dehydrogenase (G6PD) deficiency is an important public health problem, which is especially dangerous in the context of prematurity, as reflected in the US Registry. Not only is there need for better ways to identify and protect G6PD-deficient infants, but also to develop novel treatment approaches to prevent kernicterus in these infants may provide insights into preventing BIND in any jaundiced infant. Cholestasis is a problem encountered frequently in preterm infants, most often associated with intravenous feeding, and complicates the decision-making around the use of phototherapy. Finally, a practical "preemie" bilirubin toolkit is suggested as an adjunct to experience and good sense based on a sound understanding of bilirubin biochemistry and the unique vulnerabilities of the preterm infant. Although much has been written on neonatal hyperbilirubinemia, this unique issue of *Clinics in Perinatology* on hyperbilirubinemia in preterm neonates represents a focused consideration of the topic by an assembly of distinguished experts in the field.

We would like to thank Dr Ronald J. Wong for assisting with this preface.

David K. Stevenson, MD
Stanford University School of Medicine
Department of Pediatrics
Division of Neonatal and Developmental Medicine
1265 Welch Road, X157
Stanford, CA 94305, USA

Vinod K. Bhutani, MD
Stanford University School of Medicine
Department of Pediatrics
Division of Neonatal and Developmental Medicine
750 Welch Road, Suite 315
Palo Alto, CA 94304, USA

E-mail addresses:
dstevenson@stanford.edu (D.K. Stevenson)
bhutani@stanford.edu (V.K. Bhutani)

REFERENCES

1. American Academy of Pediatrics Subcommittee on Hyperbilirubinemia. Management of hyperbilirubinemia in the newborn infant 35 or more weeks of gestation. Pediatrics 2004;114:297–316.
2. Maisels MJ, Bhutani VK, Bogen D, et al. Hyperbilirubinemia in the newborn infant > or =35 weeks' gestation: an update with clarifications. Pediatrics 2009;124: 1193–8.

Hyperbilirubinemia in Preterm Neonates

Vinod K. Bhutani, MD*, Ronald J. Wong, BS, David K. Stevenson, MD

KEYWORDS

- Bilirubin • Reactive oxygen species • Photosensitivity • BIND
- Antioxidant properties

KEY POINTS

- Preterm neonates with increased bilirubin production loads are more likely to sustain adverse outcomes due to either neurotoxicity or overtreatment with phototherapy and/or exchange transfusion.
- Clinicians should rely on expert consensus opinions to guide timely and effective interventions until there is better evidence to refine bilirubin-induced neurologic dysfunction or benefits of bilirubin.
- There are clinical approaches that minimize the risk of bilirubin neurotoxicity.

INTRODUCTION

Most preterm infants less than 35 weeks gestational age (GA) have elevated total serum/plasma bilirubin (TB) levels, which often present as jaundice, the yellowish discoloration of the skin due to bilirubin deposition. When left unmonitored or untreated in these infants, an elevated TB level (hyperbilirubinemia) can progress to silent or symptomatic neurologic manifestations. Acute bilirubin encephalopathy (ABE) is acute, progressive, and often reversible with aggressive intervention, whereas kernicterus (or chronic bilirubin encephalopathy [CBE]) is the syndrome of chronic, post-icteric and permanent neurologic sequelae that is associated with more serious and usually irreversible manifestations.[1] The current management of a preterm infant with hyperbilirubinemia, who has an increased likelihood of developing bilirubin-induced neurologic damage, is under intense scrutiny. Clinicians have been instructed to use the hour-specific TB levels (Bhutani nomogram)[2] as well as considering the concurrence with the degree of an

Author Disclosure: None of the authors have financial relationships relevant to this article to disclose. None of the authors have conflicts of interest to disclose.
Division of Neonatal and Developmental Medicine, Department of Pediatrics, Stanford Children's Health, Lucile Packard Children's Hospital, Stanford University School of Medicine, Stanford, CA, USA
* Corresponding author. Department of Pediatrics, Stanford University School of Medicine, 750 Welch Road, Suite #315, Palo Alto, CA 94304.
E-mail address: bhutani@stanford.edu

Clin Perinatol 43 (2016) 215–232
http://dx.doi.org/10.1016/j.clp.2016.01.001
0095-5108/16/$ – see front matter © 2016 Elsevier Inc. All rights reserved.

infant's immaturity, illness, and/or hemolytic disease, the most common cause of increased bilirubin production, to guide the initiation of treatment. In fact, increased bilirubin production in preterm neonates adds to the risk of mortality or long-term neurodevelopmental impairment (NDI) due to bilirubin neurotoxicity[3–6] and can be manifested as the syndrome of bilirubin-induced neurologic dysfunction (BIND).[7–10] Universal screening and the prevention of Rh disease, coordinated perinatal-neonatal care, neonatal interventions with early feeding, and effective use of phototherapy has virtually eliminated the risk of kernicterus in most developed countries (ie, those with low [<5%] neonatal mortality rates).[11] Moreover, the current incidence of neurologic damage in preterm infants is also low, such that the risk-benefit spectrum for interventions should include a balance between the risk of overtreatment versus the reduction of long-term post-icteric sequelae. However, historic data attest to the increased vulnerability of the more immature neonates. In the absence of hyperbilirubinemia due to isoimmunization and without access to phototherapy or exchange transfusion (before 1955), kernicterus was reported to be 10.1%, 5.5%, and 1.2% in infants less than 30, 31 to 32, and 33 to 34 weeks GA, respectively (**Table 1**).[12] Among the infants who died due to kernicterus, 100%, 89%, 54%, and 81% were of birthweight (BW) less than 1500 g, 1500 to 2000 g, 2001 to 2500 g, and >2500 g, respectively. Overall, 60 (2.8%) of 2181 survivors of 2608 admissions to the neonatal nursery sustained kernicterus. Mortality was 73% for these 60 infants. Since 1985, phototherapy initiated at 24 ± 12 hours of life has effectively prevented hyperbilirubinemia in infants weighing less than 2000 g even in the presence of hemolysis.[12] This approach (introduced in 1985) reduced exchange transfusions from 23.9% to 4.8%. Now with 3 decades of additional experience in implementing effective phototherapy, the need for exchange transfusions has virtually been eliminated and the side effects of phototherapy in extremely low birthweight (ELBW) infants are now under active investigation. Nevertheless, bilirubin neurotoxicity continues to be associated with prematurity alone.

The ability to better predict this risk, beyond using BW and GA, has been elusive. With the known limitations of TB measurements being the ideal predictor, other biomarkers, such as unbound or "free" bilirubin (UB),[13] albumin levels, and bilirubin-albumin binding capacity (BBC), together with objective determinations of ongoing hemolysis, sepsis, and rapid rate of TB rise have been validated (**Box 1**). The individual or combined predictive utility of these measures has yet to be refined for broader

Table 1
Neonatal mortality with kernicterus among admits to neonatal nursery (by BW and GA)

GA, wk	Survivors >48 h/All NICU Admits	% Cases of Kernicterus
≥30–<31	109/264	10.1
31–32	282/356	5.7
33–34	685/801	3.2
35–36	749/792	1.1
>36	356/365	0.8
Total	2181/2608 (84%)	2.8

Abbreviations: GA, gestational age; NICU, neonatal intensive care unit.

Only sick infants >2500 g were admitted to the NICU. Neonatal risk measured in an era before the availability of phototherapy and exchange transfusion use in infants without Rh or ABO isoimmunization.

These data compare with mortality in the remainder at 23% (668/2608 NICU admissions).

Adapted from Crosse VM, Meyer TC, Gerrard JW. Kernicterus and prematurity. Arch Dis Child 1955;30:501–8.

Box 1
Historic clinical risk factors for bilirubin neurotoxicity in preterm neonates.

Clinical Risk Factors for Neurotoxicity

1. Birthweight <1000 g

2. Apgar Score <3 at 5 min of age

3. Arterial oxygen tension <40 mm Hg for >2 h

4. Arterial pH <7.15 for >1 h

5. Core temperature <35°C for >4 h

6. Serum albumin <2.5 g/dL

7. Sepsis

8. Clinical deterioration

Data from Brown AK, Kim MH, Wu PY, et al. Efficacy of phototherapy in prevention and management of neonatal hyperbilirubinemia. Pediatrics 1985;75:393–400.

---

clinical application. Immaturity, concurrent neonatal disease (such as cholestasis), and the use of total parenteral nutrition and lipid infusions (See Satrom K, Gourley G: Cholestasis in preterm infants, in this issue) or drugs that alter BBC may exacerbate the risk for BIND.[14] A clinician's treatment decisions need to be individualized for each infant and should, in general, reflect the consensus of experts, until definitive guidelines can be established. In this article, we review the evolving evidence for bilirubin-induced brain injury in preterm infants and highlight the clinical approaches that minimize the risk of bilirubin neurotoxicity.

NATURAL BILIRUBIN PROFILE IN PRETERM NEONATES

Previous studies suggest that preterm infants with modest TB levels can sustain long-term NDI at age 18 to 22 months,[7,15–18] and infants with high TB levels can experience increased mortality and NDI associated with auditory neuropathic or visuomotor processing disorders (now characterized as BIND).[7–10] However, some preterm infants are resistant to relatively high bilirubin loads in the absence of increased production rates because of efficient elimination of bilirubin and sufficient BBC.[19] Unnecessary or overprescription of phototherapy may compromise the ability of bilirubin to serve as a protective antioxidant from bilirubin neurotoxicity, which may occur at even very low TB levels.

Prevalence and Incidence

Poor correlation of visually apparent jaundice to assess hyperbilirubinemia and bilirubin neurotoxicity has confounded the accurate determination of the incidence of infants with jaundice and/or hyperbilirubinemia. It must be remembered that the degree of jaundice does not predict the TB level well. In addition, historical data on the incremental changes in clinical practice inform the evolving decline in the incidence of adverse outcomes. Prevention of Rh disease, starvation, prevention or early treatment of neonatal sepsis, safe use of antibiotics and drugs, and reduction of birth trauma have together contributed to a decrease in the incidence of kernicterus in preterm infants since the 1950s (see **Table 1**).[12] In the era before the routine use of exchange transfusion and availability of phototherapy, Crosse and colleagues[12] reported that 73.6% of preterm infants with kernicterus died compared with

25.6% for all infants born prematurely. The highest mortality rate was among those infants with lower BW and earlier age of onset of clinical signs. The sequelae or outcomes were dependent on the maturity of infants who survived the first 2 days after birth and are presented by GA stratification in **Table 1**. These data show the risk of mortality and kernicterus for preterm infants who are *not* actively treated with currently recommended strategies for treating hyperbilirubinemia. The current incidence of kernicterus in preterm infants is less certain because of highly variable implementation of bilirubin reduction strategies. In a retrospective postmortem neuropathological study,[20] the rate of kernicterus was reported to be 4% in 81 preterm infants (GA <34 weeks) who died after 48 hours of life and cared for after the introduction of phototherapy and universal Rh immunoprophylaxis. To date, there are no data on the prevalence of kernicterus in preterm survivors, but small case series of survivors with neurologic sequelae associated with hyperbilirubinemia have been reported.[4] Determining the incidence is also limited by the timeliness and aggressiveness of interventions, the variability and spectrum of BIND in preterm infants, presence of comorbidities (eg, sepsis, periventricular leukomalacia, and intraventricular hemorrhage), and delayed manifestations of hypertonicity. Clinically evident neurologic signs, such as the classic dystonic posture, dyskinesia, and abnormal muscle tone, may not manifest until 6 months corrected age. Since the late 1970s, the incidence of kernicterus in preterm infants has declined to the point where kernicterus is rarely seen postmortem, but a small number of cases of choreoathetoid cerebral palsy (CP) or sensorineural hearing loss associated with hyperbilirubinemia continue to be reported in preterm survivors.[4] The decreased incidence of kernicterus in preterm infants may, in part, be due to the initiation of proactive measures to reduce TB or to changes in neonatal care that have eliminated unappreciated risk factors for kernicterus. In a classic experiential example in a single neonatal intensive care unit (NICU), the discontinuance of bacteriostatic saline containing benzyl alcohol to flush intravenous (IV) lines led to a remarkable decline in the incidence of kernicterus from 31% to 0%.[21] Clearly, there have been dramatic improvements in the care of jaundiced preterm infants, but overall the data are sobering and still illustrate their vulnerability. Nonetheless, the reliance on a systems-approach in the NICU has led to tangible reductions in the use of exchange transfusions and of kernicterus in the United States.[22,23] It is also now well established that the presence of early-onset hyperbilirubinemia (<24 hours of age) is a medical emergency and that TB levels measured between ages 24 to 60 hours can predict the development of severe hyperbilirubinemia and an infant's need for phototherapy.[1,24] The recognition of clinical risk factors and the timeliness of interventions have probably had the most influence on neonatal outcomes.

Bilirubin Burden

The clinical burden of bilirubin neurotoxicity usually manifests as irreversible post-icteric sequelae with the hallmark sign (usually at autopsy) of icteric (yellow) staining of the basal ganglia, specifically of the globus pallidus, which can be observed as an increased signal on MRI. BIND occurs when the TB level exceeds an infant's neuroprotective defenses, primarily in the basal ganglia; central and peripheral auditory pathways; hippocampus; diencephalon; subthalamic nuclei; midbrain; pontine; brainstem nuclei for visuomotor function; respiratory, neurohumoral, and electrolyte control; and in the cerebellum, most prominently in the vermis.[23,25–28] Acute signs can present as progressive changes in an infant's cardiorespiratory status, mental (behavioral) status, and cry, with varying degrees of drowsiness, poor feeding, hypotonia, and alternating tone followed by increasing hypertonia, especially of extensor muscles, retrocollis, and opisthotonos, first intermittent and then with increasing severity, and finally becoming constant. Alternatively, clinical signs are nonspecific or absent; regardless, any neurologic sign needs to be investigated and may herald manifestations of ABE. Acute-stage mortality (about 7% in late preterm and term neonates) is due to respiratory failure and progressive coma or intractable seizures. Rate of progression of clinical signs depends on the rate of TB rise, duration of hyperbilirubinemia, host susceptibility, and presence of comorbidities. One of the more frequent morbidities is due to Rh disease (due to non-D antigens) and may manifest with fetal hydrops and lead to a complex neonatal course.

Kernicterus, often used interchangeably with CBE, is reserved for irreversible classic sequelae diagnosed in infants who survive ABE. Diagnosis is primarily dependent on presence of dystonia, athetoid CP, paralysis of upward gaze, and sensorineural hearing loss of varying degrees of severity. Cognition is usually spared to a striking degree. BIND is a wider spectrum of disorders that excludes classic (chronic) kernicterus.[8,29] Clinical evidence of damage confined to more narrow neural pathways may result in isolated, less severe clinical signs, such as auditory or visual deficits. Auditory neuropathy (or auditory "dys"-synchrony) defined by characteristic clinical criteria and distinctive findings on the auditory brainstem-evoked response (ABR) and normal cochlear function (normal cochlear microphonic, normal otoacoustic emissions [OAE]) without severe hearing loss or by similar auditory neuropathy associated with minimal fine and/or gross motor disability. Subtle neurologic manifestations of BIND include signs of awkwardness, minimal fine and gross motor incoordination, gait abnormalities, fine tremors, exaggerated extrapyramidal reflexes, and perhaps auditory learning and behavioral problems. These subtle signs are difficult to diagnose because of delayed clinical expression and their nonspecificity.

CLINICAL PROFILE OF SUBTLE POSTICTERIC SEQUELAE

As summarized by Johnson and Bhutani,[8] pilot studies conducted in the prephototherapy era for neonates cared for in 1965 to 1966, identified altered pyschometric, audiologic, speech, language, and visuomotor disorders. Their reanalysis of 4-year and 7-year follow-up studies showed a consistent, significant correlation of low bilirubin binding reserve, with suspicious and abnormal ratings for the psychometric and audiologic examinations. An abnormal bilirubin-albumin molar ratio (BAMR) appeared to predict changes in ABR. The BAMR may serve as an approximate surrogate for UB levels, and can be used as an additional factor in determining the need for exchange transfusion in neonates of 35 or more weeks GA. Preterm infants are likely to have lower serum albumin levels, and it has been suggested that the BAMR would be a good measure of the risk for bilirubin toxicity based on BW. However, its usefulness may be limited, as other factors (eg, acidosis, use of multiple drugs, elevated free fatty acids, and bilirubin photoisomers) may interfere with bilirubin-albumin binding or binding of bilirubin to sites other than albumin.[30,31]

Auditory Dysfunction

In preterm infants, the relationship between hyperbilirubinemia and hearing loss is significant and can be modulated by other risk factors.[32] Preterm infants with high TB levels ($\geq$14 mg/dL), and those with BW less than 1500 g have a higher risk of deafness than their healthy counterparts with BW more than 1500 g. Furthermore, among high-risk patients, the mean duration of hyperbilirubinemia was significantly longer in deaf infants, who appeared to have a greater number of acidotic episodes while they were hyperbilirubinemic. Hyperbilirubinemia appears to cause selective damage to the brainstem auditory nuclei and may also damage the auditory nerve and spiral ganglion.[25] In contrast, the organ of Corti and thalamocortical auditory pathways appear to be unaffected by bilirubin. Clinically, a common form of hearing loss caused by hyperbilirubinemia is auditory neuropathy spectrum disorder (ANSD).[33,34] Thus, tests of auditory transduction and outer hair cell function within the cochlea, such as the cochlear microphonics and OAEs, may be normal while ABR testing is abnormal. Some experts believe that ANSD is associated with a more subtle neurologic manifestation (BIND).[33,34] Diagnosis of ANSD is difficult due to delayed clinical onset and nonspecificity. In a study of 260 patients with ANSD, historical risk of hyperbilirubinemia was 47.7% in premature infants, and 20.3% in those who received exchange transfusion.[33] A Polish study of 9419 infants whose hearing ability was uncertain or who had risk factors for hearing loss, 352 were diagnosed with sensorineural hearing loss.[35] Of these, 18 (5.1%) were diagnosed with ANSD associated with prematurity and low BW (n = 5), pharmacologic ototoxicity (n = 8), and hyperbilirubinemia (n = 7), and 4 had no risk factors. Whether these effects are transient and have no impact on speech and language development has to yet be proven.

Visuocortical Dysfunction

Aside from the classic visuo-oculomotor manifestations of kernicterus, preliminary data have demonstrated a number of interesting and potentially worrisome findings when the visual cortex function in healthy, bilirubin-exposed infants was studied.[36] By using a quantitative measure of neural activity, the swept parameter visual-evoked potential (sVEP) response functions over a wide range of contrast, spatial frequency, and vernier offset sizes in 16 full-term infants with high TB levels (>10 mg/dL) and 18 age-matched infants with no visible neonatal jaundice, Hou and coworkers[36] compared sVEP thresholds and suprathreshold response amplitudes in all enrolled infants at 14 to 22 weeks postnatal age. Infants who had hyperbilirubinemia showed lower response amplitudes ($P<.05$) and worse or immeasurable sVEP thresholds compared with control infants for all 3 measures ($P<.05$). sVEP thresholds for vernier offset were correlated with TB levels ($P<.05$), but spatial acuity and contrast sensitivity measures in the infants with neonatal hyperbilirubinemia were not ($P>.05$). The effect of neonatal bilirubinemia on vernier acuity, which is a close surrogate for Snellen or optotype acuity, appears to be dose related. The effect of bilirubin on the visual cortex lasts well beyond the period of exposure and more than one type of vision is affected, suggesting widespread effect of bilirubin on the visual cortex.

Integrity of Brainstem Function and Structure

The frequency and distribution of periodic breathing apnea events of more than 20 seconds requiring positive pressure ventilation have been described by Amin and colleagues[37] as signs of intractable apnea and possible signs of BIND. Classic brain magnetic resonance findings for kernicterus have been reported, almost exclusively descriptive of term infants, and demonstrating vulnerability of the basal ganglia.[25] Initially, within days of a hyperbilirubinemia-related insult, T1-weighted brain imaging shows hyperintensity of the globus pallidus with or without abnormal signal in the subthalamic nuclei. Weeks or months later, T2-weighted and fluid-attenuated inversion recovery (FLAIR) images become hyperintense, and hyperintensity is no longer seen on T1-weighted images. A normal image does not eliminate the possibility of bilirubin-related brain injury; serial images may reveal an early abnormal pattern, followed by apparent resolution, then later, an abnormal T2-weighted pattern at a time that can be variable. Similarly distinctive findings have been described in a series of preterm infants of less than 30 weeks estimated gestational age (EGA).[38] In these infants, BAMRs, but not TB levels, were reported above the exchange transfusion thresholds recommended in the 1990s,[39] although all had evidence of clinical instability during their hospitalization. Therefore, it has been hypothesized that this constellation of findings may be underrecognized among preterm infants. Importantly, the bilirubin-related injury pattern can be differentiated from the most common type of preterm brain injury of white matter injury alone.[40,41]

BENEFICIAL ROLE OF BILIRUBIN

Tissue injury from a biological, chemical, or traumatic insult usually results in a cascade of adaptive response to protect against further injury possibly through restoring vascular integrity that may include endogenously elevated TB (See Stevenson DK, Wong RJ, Arnold CC, et al. Phototherapy and the risk of photo-oxidative injury in extremely low birth weight (ELBW) infants, in this issue). Mildly elevated TB may be associated with lowered morbidity and related mortality, which could be attributed to the antioxidant properties of bilirubin. The highly inducible, anti-inflammatory, antioxidant, and antiapoptotic protein, heme oxygenase-1 (HO-1) is one of the more robust mechanisms. Catalysis of the pro-oxidant heme to equimolar iron, carbon monoxide (CO), and bilirubin (converted from biliverdin) is responsible for beneficial effects of HO-1 expression to the cytoprotective properties of these by-products of the reaction. Bilirubin, generally regarded as a potentially cytotoxic, lipid-soluble waste product, is now known to exhibit potent antioxidant properties preventing the oxidative damage triggered by a wide range of oxidative stressors.[42] Therefore, the idea of a physiologic role for bilirubin in cytoprotection against short-lasting and long-lasting oxidant-mediated cell injury, such as chronic inflammatory rheumatoid arthritis, has been proposed.[43] Elevated TB levels also have been shown to be protective against stroke, atherosclerosis, and vasculitis. Earlier studies have reported negative association with coronary artery disease and possibly favorable coronary collateral growth in patients with coronary total occlusion. In another clinical example, chronic renal disease, which is associated with systemic inflammation and oxidant stress, is a strong and independent risk factor for cardiovascular disease.[44,45] Many clinical studies indicate a negative relationship of coronary artery disease as well as related mortality in patients on chronic dialysis.[46–48] A low TB concentration is associated with accelerated progression of chronic renal disease over an approximately 8-year follow-up period, indicating that bilirubin could be an independent predictor of progression.[49] Hyperbilirubinemic (>1.24 mg/dL) patients had a reduced incidence of end-stage kidney disease,[50] and that mildly elevated TB concentrations (>0.8 mg/dL) are associated with improved estimated glomerular filtration rates.[51] A negative correlation between TB concentrations and common carotid intima media thickness was reported in children who had undergone kidney transplantation and peritoneal dialysis, suggesting bilirubin may protect from vascular complications.[52] Bilirubin is also regarded as an in important multipoint inhibitor of atherosclerosis[50,53,54] and may protect from vascular damage via its antioxidant properties, thus protecting from free radical–induced damage to lipids and proteins.[55–57] Yet another example is of individuals with Gilbert syndrome who have unconjugated hyperbilirubinemia (≥1 mg/dL or 17.1 µmol/L) and whose reduced oxidative stress and inflammatory status might prevent glomerular dysfunction and vascular complications.[58] Further investigations are needed to study the protective antioxidant properties of bilirubin in sick and preterm newborns.

BENCH EVIDENCE OF BILIRUBIN NEUROTOXICITY IN PRETERM NEONATES

In a recent review, Brites and Brito[59] outlined the mechanisms of dysfunction and demise of neurons by unconjugated bilirubin (UCB) derived from excitotoxicity, oxidative stress, alterations in neuronal arborizations, synaptotoxicity, and apoptosis mediated by alterations in mitochondria dynamics and caspase activation, ultimately leading to cell demise. UCB decreases the expression of presynaptic proteins and was shown to cause presynaptic degeneration in the Gunn rat, an animal model of hyperbilirubinemia. Neurogenesis and proliferating neural stem cells and young neurons show increased susceptibility to UCB as compared with mature and old ones, thus explaining the increased vulnerability of premature infants. Neurons damaged by UCB seem less able to recover. Hippocampal neurons have shown a particular susceptibility to UCB when compared with those from cortex and cerebellum. Moreover, the addition of proinflammatory cytokines, such as tumor necrosis factor-α plus interleukin-1β, to UCB increasingly activate intracellular signaling pathways that culminate in the demise of immature neurons, providing supportive evidence for the higher risk of hyperbilirubinemia when associated with inflammation and prematurity. Hansen[60] and Watchko and Tiribelli[61] recently summarized the clinical, scientific evidence, and mechanism(s) of bilirubin neurotoxicity. These indicate that bilirubin kills specific neurons by causing necrosis; in vitro studies show that it induces apoptosis and support in vivo observations in older literature showing neuro-anatomic changes consistent with apoptosis. Evidence also suggests that bilirubin interferes with intracellular calcium homeostasis through alterations in the function and expression of calcium/calmodulin kinase II, by selectively decreasing calcium-binding proteins in susceptible brainstem areas and increasing intracellular calcium in cultured neurons, and by sensitizing the cell to other injuries or triggering apoptosis. Bilirubin also may be cytotoxic by causing neuronal hyperexcitability, perhaps via excitatory amino acid neurotoxicity, or it may have other membrane of neurotransmitter effects. Finally, it may act by interfering with mitochondrial respiration and energy production. Thus, interventions that reduce bilirubin exposure to the neonatal brain have been shown to prevent bilirubin neurotoxicity.

Prematurity in the presence of concurrent inflammatory responses in the preterm developing brain can lead to myelination delay. The initial impact on the microglial cells reacting to perinatal brain injury is by releasing proinflammatory cytokines and enhancing phagocytic potential. Thus, microglia operating during synapse formation and maturation may be dysfunctional and worsen the long-term effects on neural circuitry. In addition, astrocytic and microglial activation have been implicated in increased susceptibility to seizures, and to neurologic effects in adulthood of early-life seizures. In recent years, activated microglia have been implicated in the pathogenesis of white matter injury, such as periventricular leukomalacia.[59]

MARGINS OF CLINICAL SAFETY

Management of hyperbilirubinemia in preterm infants varies among institutions, with little evidentiary support for these differences in management.[62] Because of the limited specificity of TB as a predictor for neurotoxicity, the margin of safety is narrow and unpredictable. Thus, interventions are primarily for prevention rather than for rescue. Interventions include the following: (1) alterations of preterm gut physiology and enterohepatic circulation by early initiation of feeds to alter luminal milieu and promote gastrointestinal motility; (2) use of effective phototherapy, including irradiance and light source, as well as method and risks of exchange transfusion (not reviewed here and have been the subject of several recent reports); and (3) acute reduction of bilirubin load. Chemoprevention remains a potential option, but is limited by evidence of safety and efficacy.[63]

Recent recommendations for management of hyperbilirubinemia presented in this article (**Fig. 1**) are consensus-based. Long-term follow-up data and future randomized

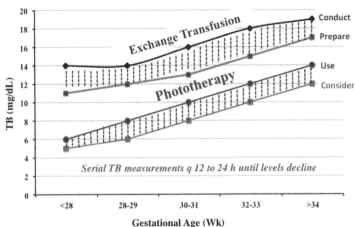

Fig. 1. Suggested use of phototherapy and exchange transfusion in preterm infants less than 35 weeks GA. The operational thresholds have been demarcated by recommendations of an expert panel. The shaded bands represent the degree of uncertainty. Recommended thresholds to prepare for exchange transfusion assume that these infants are already being managed by effective phototherapy. Increase in exposure of body surface area to phototherapy may inform the decision to conduct an exchange transfusion based on patient response to phototherapy. (*Adapted from* Maisels MJ, Watchko JF, Bhutani VK, et al. An approach to the management of hyperbilirubinemia in the preterm infant less than 35 weeks of gestation. J Perinatol 2012;32:660–4; with permission.)

controlled clinical trials may help to determine if these guidelines produce the best outcomes for preterm infants. There is a delicate balance between risk of BIND and overtreatment (and possibly, mortality) in the setting of reducing the potential antioxidant properties of bilirubin that needs more study. In the meantime, continued assessment of best practices would be helpful to minimize overtreatment or unintended consequences of bilirubin reduction strategies.

CLINICAL CARE STRATEGIES
Timing of Interventions to Reduce Excessive Bilirubin Load

The timing of bilirubin reduction strategies impacts the outcome of preterm infants at risk for excessive hyperbilirubinemia. Early implementation of strategies to rapidly and effectively reduce the excessive bilirubin load before the onset of neurologic signs, in all likelihood, could prevent chronic posticteric sequelae or kernicterus. The initial evidence for this approach, using phototherapy, was demonstrated by a National Institute of Child Health and Development (NICHD) Neonatal Research Network trial to test the efficacy of phototherapy as compared with exchange transfusion alone.[64] This study showed that phototherapy initiated at 24 ± 12 hours effectively prevented hyperbilirubinemia in infants weighing less than 2000 g even in the presence of hemolysis and reduced exchange transfusions from 23.9% to 4.8% (**Table 2**). Now, with 3 decades of experience in implementing and refining effective phototherapy, the need for exchange transfusions has virtually been eliminated. Once the clinical signs of bilirubin neurotoxicity are evident, emergent intervention to reduce the bilirubin load is the only known recourse in clinical practice. To date, exchange transfusion coupled

Table 2
Estimated risk thresholds for UB (using peroxidase assay) and calculated BBC (% saturation)

Study: (Duration/Exposure Not Measured)	UB, nM	% Saturation of BBC, Calculated
Hypothetical model[19]	20	67
Historical review[77]	17–23	63–69
Clinical: ABR changes[78]	19–33 (23)	66–77 (69)
Transient ABR changes[79]	>8.5	>46
Overt BIND[79]	>17	>63
Kernicterus present[80]	>27	>73
Kernicterus absent[80]	<13	<57
Kernicterus present[81]	>18	>65
Kernicterus absent[81]	<11	<52

Abbreviations: ABR, auditory brainstem-evoked response; BBC, bilirubin-albumin binding capacity; BIND, bilirubin-induced neurologic dysfunction; UB, unbound bilirubin.

with a "crash-cart" phototherapy remains the only known clinical option. Even though there is no predictive evidence that a specific TB level will or will not cause neurotoxic damage, the critical TB level is influenced by postnatal age, maturity, duration of hyperbilirubinemia, and rate of TB rise.

Triage for a Jaundiced Preterm Newborn with Suspicious Clinical Neurologic Signs

The triage process should be guided by ongoing staff education and development and sharing local protocols and plans of action:

1. Supplies
   Ready access to devices, equipment, and transport isolettes to manage cardio-respiratory deterioration. Specific devices include phototherapy equipment, irradiance meters specific for the device that is being used, and protective gear for the baby including opaque eye masks and filters to exclude ultraviolet light exposure. Infants with hydrops secondary to isoimmunization will likely require intensive resuscitation, stabilization, correction of anemia, and possible preparation for exchange transfusion.
2. Testing
   Transcutaneous bilirubin testing, clinical and rapid neurologic examination, and "STAT" laboratory studies (total and conjugated bilirubin and serum albumin measurements, blood typing, and cross-matching). Calculated BAMR may be assessed for additional insight to plan interventions in moderately preterm infants (**Fig. 2**). Serial bilirubin levels will need to be monitored to assess the rate of TB rise (mg/dL/h) to concurrent interventions.
3. Advise parents of the medical emergency and seek informed consent, as needed.
4. Transfer to facility that specializes in care of sick preterm neonates or commence treatment with effective phototherapy as soon as possible (crash-cart approach).

Emergency Interventions for Rapid Reduction of Bilirubin Concentrations

Rapid bilirubin reduction strategies to reverse the rapid rate of TB rise include effective phototherapy (nearly the entire body surface area [>80%]), double-volume blood exchange transfusion, and occasional need for pharmacologic agents often used in

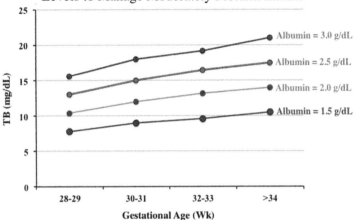

Fig. 2. Recommended use of BAMR for initiation of exchange transfusions. BAMR values have been calculated to bilirubin (mg/dL)/albumin (g/dL). Values above the thresholds for select serum albumin values of 1.5, 2.0, 2.5, and 3.0 g/dL are presented as bands above which bilirubin is likely to be displaced and may be neurotoxic. (*Data from* Ahlfors CE. Criteria for exchange transfusion in jaundiced newborns. Pediatrics 1994;93:488–94.)

combination. Effective phototherapy is the current "drug" of choice to reduce the severity of neonatal unconjugated hyperbilirubinemia (regardless of etiology) in a matter of 2 to 4 hours. Optimum use of phototherapy has been defined by specific ranges of TB thresholds that have been correlated to an infant's postnatal age (in hours) and their potential risk for bilirubin neurotoxicity (see previously). Effective phototherapy implies its use as a drug with specific light wavelengths at a specific narrow peak (460 nm, blue) and a range of emission spectrum (that is minimized from the traditional range of 400–520 nm), preferably in a precise (narrow) bandwidth that is delivered at an irradiance (dose) of greater than or equal to 25 to 30 $\mu W/cm^2/nm$ (measured specifically for the selected light wavelength) to 80% of an infant's body surface area.[65,66] There are several commercial devices and delivery methods for phototherapy for use at both the hospital and home. Blue light-emitting diodes in the 425 to 475 nm range should be easily and rapidly accessible, and periodically inspected and maintained to ensure proper functioning. Shadows with multiple lights should be avoided. The efficacy is additionally influenced by the following: (1) optimization of light administration to achieve a minimum distance between the device and the patient such that the footprint of light covers maximum surface area with minimal physical barriers; (2) infant characteristics, such as the severity of jaundice, surface area proportions, as well as dermal thickness, pigmentation, and perfusion; and (3) the duration of treatment to a specific TB threshold.[65,66]

Exchange transfusion is a critical and invasive procedure that can significantly reduce TB levels in a matter of 1 to 2 hours. Trained personnel in neonatal/pediatric intensive care facilities with full monitoring and resuscitation capabilities should perform this procedure. Exchange transfusion should be considered and anticipated when there are any neurologic signs even if TB is falling, or there are significant concerns of neurotoxicity. Concerns for neurotoxicity in term infants are heightened in an asymptomatic infant when (1) TB level exceeds 25 mg/dL; (2) intensive phototherapy fails to produce a significant TB reduction in an infant with severe hyperbilirubinemia (a progressive TB decline of at least >0.5 mg/dL per hour or >2 mg/dL drop in 4 hours should be expected) without onset of neurologic signs; or (3) an infant who had an earlier successful hearing screen and fails an automated ABR screen. Before an exchange transfusion is initiated, the health care team should review the risks and benefits of the procedure with the parents, so parents can provide informed parental consent (see later in this article). The adverse effects of an exchange transfusion include neonatal morbidities such as apnea, anemia, thrombocytopenia, electrolyte and calcium imbalances, risk of necrotizing enterocolitis, hemorrhage, infection, complications related to the use of blood products, and catheter-related complications.[67] Exchange transfusion also carries the risk of neonatal mortality, especially in sick infants. Exchange transfusion is ideally performed as an isovolumic procedure, preferably with concurrent withdrawal from an arterial line and infusion through a venous line. Double-volume exchange (170 mL/kg) is preferable, but in the event of technical difficulties, a single-volume exchange transfusion may be adequate if supplemented with intensive phototherapy. The entire process should be accomplished within 4 to 6 hours of the identification of the medical emergency.[1] Pharmacologic options and chemoprevention strategies have been reviewed in recent articles,[63,68] but have a limited role in the emergency room management of a sick infant.

Albumin Infusion

At times, an albumin infusion (1 g/kg) has been suggested before an exchange transfusion, especially if serum albumin is low (<3.0 g/dL).[69] However, there is no current evidence to support this practice. In the preterm infant, there is concern for increased intravascular volume, increased alveolar leak, and cardiopulmonary compromise.

Intravenous Gamma Immunoglobulin

Intravenous gamma immunoglobulin (IVIG) may be administered when the hyperbilirubinemia is attributed to isoimmunization. IVIG has been shown, anecdotally, to reduce the need for exchange transfusions in Rh and ABO hemolytic diseases.[1,70,71] Although data are limited, there is no evidentiary basis for its use and there are concerns for significant side effects in preterm neonates.

Phenobarbital

Phenobarbital can accelerate bilirubin excretion by increasing hepatic clearance.[71] However, this drug is no longer recommended, as it has no clinical effect when administered to infants of less than 32 weeks GA and is ineffective when given before 12 hours of age. The adverse effects of this therapy include sedation, risk of hemorrhagic disease, and the potentially addictive nature of phenobarbital.[72] This drug has a slow onset of effect (usually several days) and a long duration of action (1–2 weeks) after its discontinuation. For all of these reasons, the use of phenobarbital is no longer recommended.

Metalloporphyrins

Synthetic heme analogs or metalloporphyrins can inhibit HO, the rate-limiting enzyme in the bilirubin production pathway.[73] Some have been noted to cause photosensitization (especially during exposure to intense fluorescent light). These drugs are being investigated in clinical pharmacologic and toxicologic studies and have been shown to reduce TB levels.[63,74] The Food and Drug Administration has not yet approved their use in the United States.

Other strategies that warrant further investigations and clinical trials are use of agents that interrupt the enterohepatic circulation and bilirubin accumulation from the continued action of β-glucuronidase. Chemoprevention with use of casein supplements or other agents, such as L-aspartic acid, could decrease intestinal reabsorption of bilirubin and may play a potential preventive or adjunctive clinical role.[75]

FOLLOW-UP OF PRETERM INFANTS AT RISK FOR BILIRUBIN-INDUCED NEUROLOGIC DYSFUNCTION

Posticteric sequelae are often unrecognized, mislabeled, or misdiagnosed in preterm infants. These errors have led to prolonged diagnostic and health-seeking odysseys for families. Follow-up studies of infants enrolled in the NICHD trial of 1979 to 1985 demonstrated the challenges of follow-up in this population as well as the residual morbidities identified at late childhood and in adults. Oh and colleagues,[16] through a retrospective observational analysis in infants with BW less than 1000 g, noted that TB concentrations during the first 14 days of birth are directly correlated with death, NDI, sensorineural hearing loss, and other physical impairments. Confounding effects of modest hyperbilirubinemia or potential toxic effects of phototherapy could not be excluded.[16] These have been supplemented by similar concerns for adverse outcomes at age 16 to 22 months for preterm infants weighing less than 1000 g.[76] Infants with TB levels that approach thresholds for an exchange transfusion should be followed through infancy until school age for awkwardness, gait abnormality, failure of fine stereognosis, gaze abnormalities, poor coordination, and exaggerated extrapyramidal reflexes. Follow-up should include neurologic and neurodevelopmental evaluation, neuroimaging with magnetic resonance, and ABRs.

SUMMARY

Bilirubin, a powerful antioxidant, also can act as a powerful but silent neurotoxin at the most vulnerable stage of preterm life. The impact is long-lasting with both functional and structural neurologic injury that alters the processing of afferent input and leads to disordered efferent function. Moreover, these perturbations can potentially arrest or retard the natural neural maturation and/or lead to disordered clinical extrapyramidal function, sensory processing of hearing, visual responses, and learning. At a cellular level, development of neurogenic niches and maturation of both vascular endothelial cells and glial cells are significant in the immediate postnatal period, which may be amplified by the concomitant stresses that can accompany these exposures, such as prematurity, inflammation/sepsis, and oxidative stress. Innovative rehabilitation techniques during early follow-up may promote plastic compensation for loss of function. Functional recovery would depend on the ability of the maturing brain to reestablish neuroplasticity as with most preterm neonates at risk for developmental sequelae. In the future, advances in neuroimaging techniques, comprehensive evaluation for the integrity of auditory and visual responses, and specific testing for extrapyramidal neuromotor performances may contribute to the increased recognition of bilirubin-related neurologic sequelae. In the meantime, as better predictive biomarkers are validated, individualized clinical judgment is the key to balance the risks and benefits of preventive, effective, and timely interventions.

Best practices

What is the current practice?

To reduce the bilirubin load and use of exchange transfusion in preterm infants.

Current practices include the following:
- Early onset of enteral feeding
- Proactive use of effective phototherapy
- Clinical reliance on TB levels to assess bilirubin load
- Identification of vulnerable infants with hemolysis, sepsis, or hypoalbuminemia

Best practice recommendations

- Use consensus and expert recommendations for initiation and use of phototherapy until predictive evidence is validated in prospective studies
- Minimize, based on clinical judgment, exposure to phototherapy in ELBW infants who may be more vulnerable to side effects of photo-oxidant injury, yet more at risk for developing bilirubin-related neurotoxicity if left untreated
- Aggressive reduction of bilirubin load if there is onset of any neurologic signs
- Be informed of hypoalbuminemia or any concurrent conditions that may alter bilirubin binding to albumin and increase the potential risk of BIND

What changes in current practice are likely to improve outcomes?

- Research regarding proven predictive biomarkers of BIND
- Early recognition of rate of rise in TB levels that could overwhelm the bilirubin binding to albumin in preterm neonates
- Consistent use of blue light-emitting diode devices to deliver phototherapy and implement the American Academy of Pediatrics guideline
- Develop quality improvement measures that promote use of phototherapy as a "drug"

Is there a clinical algorithm?

- See **Figs. 1** and **2** algorithms that guide interventions using expert recommendations.

Summary statement

Hyperbilirubinemia in preterm infants is related to increased bilirubin production and/or concurrent delayed bilirubin elimination. Clinical burden of hyperbilirubinemia is confounded by an infant's prematurity, delayed enteral feeding, presence of neonatal sepsis, use of drugs that impede bilirubin binding to albumin, and cholestasis that is often attributed to prolonged use of parenteral nutrition. A higher risk of mortality, long-term neurologic injury, and risk of subtle sequelae (BIND) have been more evident in preterm as compared with term neonates. Evaluation of bilirubin load includes determination of TB, rate of rise of TB for age in hours, serum albumin levels, UB, and BBC, as well as measures of bilirubin production (such as end-tidal carbon monoxide, corrected for ambient CO (ETCOc) or carboxyhemoglobin, corrected for ambient CO [COHbc]). Early enteral feeding and optimization of narrow-band light wavelength phototherapy are the current ways to prevent and treat progressive hyperbilirubinemia in newborns less than 35 weeks of GA. Effective and widely accessible phototherapy has resulted in rare occurrences of ABE and CBE as well as the infrequent need for exchange transfusion. However, recently there are more reports of potential for photo-oxidant injury in the management of ELBW infants exposed to phototherapy.

REFERENCES

1. American Academy of Pediatrics. Management of hyperbilirubinemia in the newborn infant 35 or more weeks of gestation. Pediatrics 2004;114:297–316.
2. Bhutani VK, Johnson L, Sivieri EM. Predictive ability of a predischarge hour-specific serum bilirubin for subsequent significant hyperbilirubinemia in healthy term and near-term newborns. Pediatrics 1999;103:6–14.

3. Johnson L, Bhutani VK, Karp K, et al. Clinical report from the pilot USA kernicterus registry (1992 to 2004). J Perinatol 2009;29(Suppl 1):S25–45.
4. Bhutani VK, Johnson LH, Shapiro SM. Kernicterus in sick and preterm infants (1999-2002): a need for an effective preventive approach. Semin Perinatol 2004;28:319–25.
5. Bhutani VK, Vilms RJ, Hamerman-Johnson L. Universal bilirubin screening for severe neonatal hyperbilirubinemia. J Perinatol 2010;30(Suppl):S6–15.
6. Watchko JF, Oski FA. Kernicterus in preterm newborns: past, present, and future. Pediatrics 1992;90:707–15.
7. Broman SH, Nicholas PI, Kennedy WA. Preschool IQ: prenatal and early developmental correlates. Hillsdale (NJ): Lawrence Erlbaum Associates; 1975.
8. Johnson L, Bhutani VK. The clinical syndrome of bilirubin-induced neurologic dysfunction. Semin Perinatol 2011;35:101–13.
9. Scheidt PC, Graubard BI, Nelson KB, et al. Intelligence at six years in relation to neonatal bilirubin levels: follow-up of the National Institute of Child Health and Human Development Clinical Trial of Phototherapy. Pediatrics 1991;87:797–805.
10. Bhutani VK, Wong RJ. Bilirubin-induced neurologic dysfunction. Semin Fetal Neonatal Med 2015;20:1–64.
11. Bhutani VK, Zipursky A, Blencowe H, et al. Neonatal hyperbilirubinemia and Rhesus disease of the newborn: incidence and impairment estimates for 2010 at regional and global levels. Pediatr Res 2013;74(Suppl 1):86–100.
12. Crosse VM, Meyer TC, Gerrard JW. Kernicterus and prematurity. Arch Dis Child 1955;30:501–8.
13. Oh W, Stevenson DK, Tyson JE, et al. Influence of clinical status on the association between plasma total and unbound bilirubin and death or adverse neurodevelopmental outcomes in extremely low birth weight infants. Acta Paediatr 2010; 99:673–8.
14. Brodersen R. Competitive binding of bilirubin and drugs to human serum albumin studied by enzymatic oxidation. J Clin Invest 1974;54:1353–64.
15. Morris BH, Oh W, Tyson JE, et al. Aggressive vs. conservative phototherapy for infants with extremely low birth weight. N Engl J Med 2008;359:1885–96.
16. Oh W, Tyson JE, Fanaroff AA, et al. Association between peak serum bilirubin and neurodevelopmental outcomes in extremely low birth weight infants. Pediatrics 2003;112:773–9.
17. O'Shea TM, Dillard RG, Klinepeter KL, et al. Serum bilirubin levels, intracranial hemorrhage, and the risk of developmental problems in very low birth weight neonates. Pediatrics 1992;90:888–92.
18. Yeo KL, Perlman M, Hao Y, et al. Outcomes of extremely premature infants related to their peak serum bilirubin concentrations and exposure to phototherapy. Pediatrics 1998;102:1426–31.
19. Lamola AA, Bhutani VK, Du L, et al. Neonatal bilirubin binding capacity discerns risk of neurological dysfunction. Pediatr Res 2015;77:334–9.
20. Ahdab-Barmada M, Moossy J. The neuropathology of kernicterus in the premature neonate: diagnostic problems. J Neuropathol Exp Neurol 1984;43:45–56.
21. Jardine DS, Rogers K. Relationship of benzyl alcohol to kernicterus, intraventricular hemorrhage, and mortality in preterm infants. Pediatrics 1989;83:153–60.
22. Bhutani VK, Johnson LH, Jeffrey Maisels M, et al. Kernicterus: epidemiological strategies for its prevention through systems-based approaches. J Perinatol 2004;24:650–62.
23. Johnson LH, Bhutani VK, Brown AK. System-based approach to management of neonatal jaundice and prevention of kernicterus. J Pediatr 2002;140:396–403.

24. Bhutani VK, Stark AR, Lazzeroni LC, et al. Predischarge screening for severe neonatal hyperbilirubinemia identifies infants who need phototherapy. J Pediatr 2013;162:477–82.e1.

25. Shapiro SM. Chronic bilirubin encephalopathy: diagnosis and outcome. Semin Fetal Neonatal Med 2010;15:157–63.

26. Perlstein M. Neurologic sequelae of erythroblastosis fetalis. Am J Dis Child 1950; 79:605–6.

27. Van Praagh R. Diagnosis of kernicterus in the neonatal period. Pediatrics 1961; 28:870–6.

28. Volpe JJ. Bilirubin and brain injury. In: Volpe JJ, editor. Neurology of the newborn. 2nd edition. Philadelphia: W.B. Saunders; 2000. p. 490–514.

29. Bhutani VK, Wong RJ. Bilirubin neurotoxicity in preterm infants: risk and prevention. J Clin Neonatol 2013;2:61–9.

30. Brodersen R, Stern L. Deposition of bilirubin acid in the central nervous system–a hypothesis for the development of kernicterus. Acta Paediatr Scand 1990;79:12–9.

31. Walker PC. Neonatal bilirubin toxicity. A review of kernicterus and the implications of drug-induced bilirubin displacement. Clin Pharmacokinet 1987;13:26–50.

32. De Vries LS, Lary S, Whitelaw AG, et al. Relationship of serum bilirubin levels and hearing impairment in newborn infants. Early Hum Dev 1987;15:269–77.

33. Berlin CI, Hood LJ, Morlet T, et al. Multi-site diagnosis and management of 260 patients with auditory neuropathy/dys-synchrony (auditory neuropathy spectrum disorder). Int J Audiol 2010;49:30–43.

34. Chisin R, Perlman M, Sohmer H. Cochlear and brain stem responses in hearing loss following neonatal hyperbilirubinemia. Ann Otol 1979;88:352–7.

35. Bielecki I, Horbulewicz A, Wolan T. Prevalence and risk factors for auditory neuropathy spectrum disorder in a screened newborn population at risk for hearing loss. Int J Pediatr Otorhinolaryngol 2012;76:1668–70.

36. Hou C, Norcia AM, Madan A, et al. Visuocortical function in infants with a history of neonatal jaundice. Invest Ophthalmol Vis Sci 2014;55:6443–9.

37. Amin SB, Bhutani VK, Watchko JF. Apnea in acute bilirubin encephalopathy. Semin Perinatol 2014;38:407–11.

38. Govaert P, Lequin M, Swarte R, et al. Changes in globus pallidus with (pre)term kernicterus. Pediatrics 2003;112:1256–63.

39. Ahlfors CE. Criteria for exchange transfusion in jaundiced newborns. Pediatrics 1994;93:488–94.

40. Khwaja O, Volpe JJ. Pathogenesis of cerebral white matter injury of prematurity. Arch Dis Child Fetal Neonatal Ed 2008;93:F153–61.

41. Rutherford MA, Supramaniam V, Ederies A, et al. Magnetic resonance imaging of white matter diseases of prematurity. Neuroradiology 2010;52:505–21.

42. Stocker R, Yamamoto Y, McDonagh AF, et al. Bilirubin is an antioxidant of possible physiological importance. Science 1987;235:1043–6.

43. Fischman D, Valluri A, Gorrepati VS, et al. Bilirubin as a protective factor for rheumatoid arthritis: an NHANES study of 2003-2006 data. J Clin Med Res 2010;2: 256–60.

44. Takamatsu N, Abe H, Tominaga T, et al. Risk factors for chronic kidney disease in Japan: a community-based study. BMC Nephrol 2009;10:34.

45. Yamamoto R, Kanazawa A, Shimizu T, et al. Association between atherosclerosis and newly classified chronic kidney disease stage for Japanese patients with type 2 diabetes. Diabetes Res Clin Pract 2009;84:39–45.

46. Chen YH, Hung SC, Tarng DC. Serum bilirubin links UGT1A1*28 polymorphism and predicts long-term cardiovascular events and mortality in chronic hemodialysis patients. Clin J Am Soc Nephrol 2011;6:567–74.
47. Fukui M, Tanaka M, Yamazaki M, et al. Low serum bilirubin concentration in haemodialysis patients with type 2 diabetes. Diabet Med 2011;28:96–9.
48. Riphagen IJ, Deetman PE, Bakker SJ, et al. Bilirubin and progression of nephropathy in type 2 diabetes: a post hoc analysis of RENAAL with independent replication in IDNT. Diabetes 2014;63:2845–53.
49. Tanaka M, Fukui M, Okada H, et al. Low serum bilirubin concentration is a predictor of chronic kidney disease. Atherosclerosis 2014;234:421–5.
50. Oda E, Aoyagi R, Aizawa Y. Hypobilirubinemia might be a possible risk factor of end-stage kidney disease independently of estimated glomerular filtration rate. Kidney Blood Press Res 2012;36:47–54.
51. Chin HJ, Cho HJ, Lee TW, et al. The mildly elevated serum bilirubin level is negatively associated with the incidence of end stage renal disease in patients with IgA nephropathy. J Korean Med Sci 2009;24(Suppl):S22–9.
52. Dvorakova HM, Szitanyi P, Dvorak P, et al. Determinants of premature atherosclerosis in children with end-stage renal disease. Physiol Res 2012;61:53–61.
53. Boon AC, Bulmer AC, Coombes JS, et al. Circulating bilirubin and defense against kidney disease and cardiovascular mortality: mechanisms contributing to protection in clinical investigations. Am J Physiol Renal Physiol 2014;307: F123–36.
54. Wagner KH, Wallner M, Molzer C, et al. Looking to the horizon: the role of bilirubin in the development and prevention of age-related chronic diseases. Clin Sci (Lond) 2015;129:1–25.
55. Bulmer AC, Blanchfield JT, Toth I, et al. Improved resistance to serum oxidation in Gilbert's syndrome: a mechanism for cardiovascular protection. Atherosclerosis 2008;199:390–6.
56. Neuzil J, Stocker R. Free and albumin-bound bilirubin are efficient co-antioxidants for alpha-tocopherol, inhibiting plasma and low density lipoprotein lipid peroxidation. J Biol Chem 1994;269:16712–9.
57. Stocker R, Peterhans E. Antioxidant properties of conjugated bilirubin and biliverdin: biologically relevant scavenging of hypochlorous acid. Free Radic Res Commun 1989;6:57–66.
58. do Sameiro-Faria M, Kohlova M, Ribeiro S, et al. Potential cardiovascular risk protection of bilirubin in end-stage renal disease patients under hemodialysis. Biomed Res Int 2014;2014:175286.
59. Brites D, Brito A. Bilirubin toxicity. In: Stevenson DK, Maisels MJ, Watchko JF, editors. Neonatal jaundice. New York: The McGraw Hill Companies; 2012. p. 115–43.
60. Hansen TW. Prevention of neurodevelopmental sequelae of jaundice in the newborn. Dev Med Child Neurol 2011;53(Suppl 4):24–8.
61. Watchko JF, Tiribelli C. Bilirubin-induced neurologic damage. N Engl J Med 2014; 370:979.
62. Maisels MJ, Watchko JF, Bhutani VK, et al. An approach to the management of hyperbilirubinemia in the preterm infant less than 35 weeks of gestation. J Perinatol 2012;32:660–4.
63. Schulz S, Wong RJ, Vreman HJ, et al. Metalloporphyrins—an update. Front Pharmacol 2012;3:68.
64. Brown AK, Kim MH, Wu PY, et al. Efficacy of phototherapy in prevention and management of neonatal hyperbilirubinemia. Pediatrics 1985;75:393–400.

65. Vreman HJ, Wong RJ, Stevenson DK. Phototherapy: current methods and future directions. Semin Perinatol 2004;28:326–33.

66. Bhutani VK, Fetus and Newborn, American Academy of Pediatrics. Phototherapy to prevent severe neonatal hyperbilirubinemia in the newborn infant 35 or more weeks of gestation. Pediatrics 2011;128:e1046–52.

67. Murki S, Kumar P. Blood exchange transfusion for infants with severe neonatal hyperbilirubinemia. Semin Perinatol 2011;35:175–84.

68. Drummond GS, Kappas A. Chemoprevention of severe neonatal hyperbilirubinemia. Semin Perinatol 2004;28:365–8.

69. Maisels MJ, Bhutani VK, Bogen D, et al. Hyperbilirubinemia in the newborn infant > or =35 weeks' gestation: an update with clarifications. Pediatrics 2009; 124:1193–8.

70. Rübo J, Albrecht K, Lasch P, et al. High-dose intravenous immune globulin therapy for hyperbilirubinemia caused by Rh hemolytic disease. J Pediatr 1992;121:93–7.

71. Okuda H, Potter BJ, Blades B, et al. Dose-related effects of phenobarbital on hepatic glutathione-S-transferase activity and ligandin levels in the rat. Drug Metab Dispos 1989;17:677–82.

72. Wallin A, Boreus LO. Phenobarbital prophylaxis for hyperbilirubinemia in preterm infants. A controlled study of bilirubin disappearance and infant behavior. Acta Paediatr Scand 1984;73:488–97.

73. Tenhunen R, Marver HS, Schmid R. The enzymatic conversion of heme to bilirubin by microsomal heme oxygenase. Proc Natl Acad Sci U S A 1968;61:748–55.

74. Wong RJ, Vreman HJ, Schulz S, et al. In vitro inhibition of heme oxygenase isoenzymes by metalloporphyrins. J Perinatol 2011;31(Suppl 1):S35–41.

75. Gourley GR. Breast-feeding, neonatal jaundice and kernicterus. Semin Neonatol 2002;7:135–41.

76. Hintz SR, Stevenson DK, Yao Q, et al. Is phototherapy exposure associated with better or worse outcomes in 501- to 1000-g-birth-weight infants? Acta Paediatr 2011;100:960–5.

77. Ahlfors CE, Wennberg RP, Ostrow JD, et al. Unbound (free) bilirubin: improving the paradigm for evaluating neonatal jaundice. Clin Chem 2009;55:1288–99.

78. Funato M, Tamai H, Shimada S, et al. Vigintiphobia, unbound bilirubin, and auditory brainstem responses. Pediatrics 1994;93:50–3.

79. Amin SB, Ahlfors C, Orlando MS, et al. Bilirubin and serial auditory brainstem responses in premature infants. Pediatrics 2001;107:664–70.

80. Cashore WJ, Oh W. Unbound bilirubin and kernicterus in low-birth-weight infants. Pediatrics 1982;69:481–5.

81. Ritter DA, Kenny JD, Norton HJ, et al. A prospective study of free bilirubin and other risk factors in the development of kernicterus in premature infants. Pediatrics 1982;69:260–6.

Hemolysis in Preterm Neonates

Robert D. Christensen, MD[a,b,*], Hassan M. Yaish, MD[a]

KEYWORDS

- Bilirubin • Anemia • Prematurity • End-tidal carbon monoxide • Haptoglobin
- Next-generation DNA sequencing

KEY POINTS

- Identifying hemolysis in premature neonates can be more difficult than in term neonates; recommendations for identifying hemolysis are presented.
- When hemolysis is recognized in a premature neonate, caregivers should be alerted to the possibility of (1) a relatively rapid rise in total serum/plasma bilirubin, (2) hyperbilirubinemia that is relatively slow to abate with phototherapy, and (3) hyperbilirubinemia that is likely to rebound after phototherapy is discontinued.
- The bilirubin load a preterm neonate receives from a donor red blood cell transfusion is influenced by the percentage of donor cells lysed during storage before the transfusion.
- The genetic conditions that cause hemolytic jaundice in term neonates, such as erythrocyte cytoskeletal protein mutations and enzymatic defects, also occur in premature neonates.

WHAT IS HEMOLYSIS?

When erythrocytes emerge from the marrow (or, in preterm infants, from the liver and the marrow) into the blood, they typically remain in circulation for a certain number of days. This length of time is known as the red blood cell (RBC) life span.[1,2] In adults, the RBC life span is 100 to 120 days.[3,4] In term neonates, it is approximately 60 to 80 days.[5] In preterm infants, the RBC life span is shorter still and is likely shorter in

Disclosures: Dr R.D. Christensen is an uncompensated advisor to Capnia Inc, Redwood Shores, CA, USA. Both Drs R.D. Christensen and H.M. Yaish served as uncompensated advisors to ARUP Laboratories, Salt Lake City, UT, USA, testing Band 3 reduction for diagnosing hereditary spherocytosis in neonates and the 28-gene next-generation sequencing panel for identifying genetic causes of otherwise unexplained neonatal jaundice.

[a] Division of Hematology/Oncology, Department of Pediatrics, Primary Children's Hospital, University of Utah School of Medicine, Chipeta Way, Salt Lake City, UT 84108, USA; [b] Women and Newborn's Clinical Program, Division of Neonatology, Department of Pediatrics, Intermountain Healthcare, University of Utah School of Medicine, Chipeta Way, Salt Lake City, UT 84108, USA
* Corresponding author. Department of Pediatrics, University of Utah, 295 Chipeta Way, Salt Lake City, UT 84108.
E-mail address: robert.christensen@hsc.utah.edu

Clin Perinatol 43 (2016) 233–240
http://dx.doi.org/10.1016/j.clp.2016.01.002
0095-5108/16/$ – see front matter © 2016 Elsevier Inc. All rights reserved.

proportion to gestational age (GA); however, the details of this relationship remain unclear.[3–7] The definition of hemolysis is an RBC life span significantly shorter than it should be and associated with increased bilirubin production.[1,2]

The process of natural termination of the RBC life span in circulation is a physiologic process known as senescence. In contrast, hemolysis is a pathologic shortening of the RBC life span due to a wide range of conditions, including genetically based abnormalities in RBC structure or function,[8] antibodies attached to erythrocytes leading to premature removal, or issues extrinsic to RBCs. These issues include physical disruption; injury by infectious agents, temperature, or chemicals; or injury by disruption from tethering on fibrin strands as occurs in disseminated intravascular coagulation (DIC). Extravasation of blood into tissues is another cause of hemolysis that is encountered in bruising, cephalohematoma, subgaleal hemorrhages, or intraventricular hemorrhages because the RBCs in the environment of tissues are metabolized much more rapidly than had they remained in circulation.

The consequence of any hemolytic process is bilirubin load that is larger than normal. This is because heme is metabolized to bilirubin.[9,10] Conceptually, the bilirubin load is the amount of bilirubin that must be taken up by hepatocytes, conjugated, and excreted. When hemolysis produces an excessive bilirubin load, which cannot be metabolized efficiently by normally functioning bilirubin metabolic mechanisms, the total serum/plasma bilirubin (TB) concentration rises and may result in hemolytic jaundice that could be associated with hemolytic anemia.[11–13]

When hemolysis is recognized as the cause of jaundice and/or anemia in a preterm infant, caregivers should be aware of the possibility that (1) TB can rise rapidly, (2) the hyperbilirubinemia may be somewhat slow to fall with phototherapy, and (3) the hyperbilirubinemia is more likely to rebound after phototherapy is discontinued.[9,10]

HOW IS HEMOLYSIS RECOGNIZED IN A JAUNDICED PRETERM INFANT?

In neonates, a set of laboratory tests can be used to identify the presence of a hemolytic process, although they are often limited by their individual specificity.[14] Unfortunately, when applied to preterm infants, these tests all have additional limitations compared with their use in term neonates. **Table 1** lists the tests typically used to diagnose hemolysis in infants and children, and reviews the pitfalls or problems when applying these tests to preterm neonates.

When heme is metabolized to bilirubin, equimolar amounts of carbon monoxide (CO) is generated and exhaled.[11] Therefore, measuring the end-tidal or exhaled breath CO concentration, corrected for inhaled CO (ETCOc) provides a quantitative measurement of the hemolytic rate.[11,12,15,16] It was previously reported that in term neonates the upper reference range level of ETCOc during the first week after birth is 1.7 ppm but in preterm infants this upper range value is not yet known.[15,16] Also, preterm infants might have tachypnea, and the presently available ETCOc monitor (CoSense, Capnia Inc, Redwood Shores, CA, USA) does not consistently provide data if the respiratory rate exceeds 60 breaths per minute. Also, the present instrumentation is not usable for neonates on mechanical ventilation or continuous positive airway pressure.

Many of the tests used to identify hemolysis have not been specifically validated in preterm infants. Values for reticulocytes, immature reticulocyte fraction, and nucleated RBCs are definitely different in preterm than in term neonates, and they vary with GA at birth and with postnatal age.[17,18]

Erythrocyte morphology, judged by light microscopy, is challenging in preterm infants because the erythrocytes tend to have greater percentages of abnormal forms than those found in term neonates. However, careful examination for the presence

Table 1
Tests performed on jaundiced neonates to identify a hemolytic component

Test	Reference Intervals	Problems Applying the Test to Preterm Neonates
Hemoglobinuria	≥Trace hemoglobin in urinalysis	RBCs in urine not uncommon in VLBW neonates When present, urinary hemoglobin invalid
Low or absent serum haptoglobin	A value that is falling or < the lower limit of detection	Preterm infants without hemolysis may have very low serum haptoglobin concentrations
DAT (Coombs)	Positive direct or indirect Coombs	Accuracy may be less among VLBW neonates
Elevated absolute reticulocyte count	>Upper limit for GA	Preterm infants can normally have elevated reticulocytes, according to GA
Elevated immature reticulocyte fraction	Value >7% at birth or >3% after 24 h	Not well validated in VLBW neonates
Elevated nucleated RBC count	Upper limit 3000/μL at birth Should be <500/μL after 3–4 d	Not well validated in VLBW neonates Nucleated RBCs typically higher in younger GA at birth
Abnormal RBC morphology on stained blood film	Microspherocytes, elliptocytes, bite and blister cells, echinocytes, schistocytes	Anisocytosis and poikilocytosis frequently encountered in healthy preterm neonates
Heinz body preparation	Heinz bodies support diagnosis of hemolysis due to precipitated (unstable) hemoglobin	Less well studied in preterm infants
Elevated ETCOc	First week or 2 the upper limit = 1.7–2 ppm, thereafter the upper limit = 1 ppm	Reference intervals for VLBW neonates lacking Cannot perform test if neonate intubated or on nasal cannula oxygen Difficult to get accurate reading if respiratory rate is >60 breaths/min
Carboxyhemoglobin by carbon monoxide oximetry	Upper limit = 1.5–2.0%	Reference intervals for VLBW neonates lacking Measurement not sensitive

Abbreviations: DAT, direct antiglobulin test; ETCOc, end-tidal or exhaled breath carbon monoxide concentration, corrected for inhaled carbon monoxide; VLBW, very low birth weight.

of microspherocytes, polychromatophilia, bite and blister cells, echinocytes, and schistocytes can be of significant value in suspecting hemolysis as well as in giving some clues into the cause of the hemolytic process.[19]

WHAT IS THE RISK TO A PRETERM INFANT IN WHOM A DONOR RED BLOOD CELL TRANSFUSION WILL RESULT IN A RISE IN TOTAL SERUM/PLASMA BILIRUBIN?

Many factors can exacerbate neonatal hyperbilirubinemia and thereby increase the risk for bilirubin neurotoxicity.[9–13] RBC transfusions have the potential to increase

Table 2
Estimation of the rise in total serum/plasma bilirubin following donor red blood cell transfusion as a function of the percent of donor red blood cells lysed before (or during) transfusion

Assumptions	Amount of Free Hemoglobin Transfused into the Neonate	Expected Posttransfusion Rise in TB Based On Added Bilirubin Load
1% of donor RBCs lysed	0.03 g/kg recipient	1.2 mg/dL
5% of donor RBCs lysed	0.15 g/kg recipient	6 mg/dL
10% of donor RBCs lysed	0.3 g/kg recipient	12 mg/dL

Adapted from Christensen RD, Baer VL, Snow GL. Association of neonatal red blood cell transfusion with increase in serum bilirubin. Transfusion 2014;54:3068; with permission.

the TB as a result of lysis of the banked donor RBC before, during, or after the transfusion, plus immaturity of the mechanisms involved in bilirubin metabolism, such as the physiologically low activity of bilirubin-conjugation during the early days after birth.[20]

In theory, if 1% of the transfused donor RBC lysed in a 15 mL/kg transfusion of packed RBCs, the TB would rise concurrently by approximately 1.2 mg/dL (**Table 2**). Likewise, if 10% of the donor RBC lysed, the TB would rise by 12 mg/dL. Ozment and colleagues[21] reported that hemolysis of donor RBCs increased significantly during storage time as demonstrated by increases in free hemoglobin. They quantified free hemoglobin in 12 leukoreduced RBC units obtained from the American Red Cross. The average concentration of free hemoglobin increased from 20 mg/dL after 4 days storage to about 60 mg/dL at 21 days, and to about 120 mg/dL by 42 days.

In a recent retrospective study, Christensen and colleagues[20] found that 12% of RBC transfusions to very low birth weight (VLBW) infants (<1500 g) were followed by TB increases greater than or equal to 5 mg/dL. Transfusions of neonates with universal donor blood (O negative) resulted in a higher TB rise (*P*<.0001) but the magnitude was clinically insignificant (0.3 mg/dL).

Fig. 1 shows TB levels before and within 28 hours of RBC transfusions in a neonatal intensive care unit. The largest increases in TB levels occurred when transfusions were

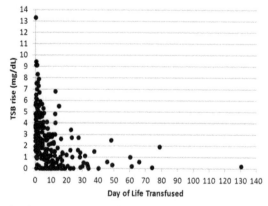

Fig. 1. The relationship between magnitude of rise in TB (following an RBC transfusion, and age of the neonate transfused (days since birth). As the neonate ages, the magnitude of rise in TB after transfusion decreases (*P*<.001). TSB, total serum bilirubin. (*Adapted from* Christensen RD, Baer VL, Snow GL. Association of neonatal red blood cell transfusion with increase in serum bilirubin. Transfusion 2014;54:3071; with permission.)

given during the first days after birth, perhaps because of immature mechanisms regulating bilirubin uptake and conjugation. Hence, RBC transfusion of premature neonates, particularly during their first days after birth, may carry some risk of hyperbilirubinemia. Usually the magnitude of TB rise is insignificant but clinicians

Table 3
The genes sequenced in a neonatal jaundice next-generation sequencing panel

Gene Symbol	Gene Description	Associated Hematological Disorder
SPTA1	Spectrin alpha	Elliptocytosis, spherocytosis, pyropoikilocytosis
SPTB	Spectrin beta	Elliptocytosis, spherocytosis
ANK1	Ankyrin 1	Spherocytosis
SLC4A1	Solute carrier family 4, anion exchanges, member 1 (erythrocyte membrane protein band 3)	Spherocytosis, stomatocytosis, acanthocytosis, ovalocytosis
EPB41	Erythrocyte membrane protein band 4.1	Elliptocytosis
EPB42	Erythrocyte membrane protein band 4.2	Spherocytosis
PIEZO1	Piezo-type mechanosensitive ion channel component 1	Xerocytosis
CYB5R3	Cytochrome b reductase 3	Methemoglobinemia type 1 & 2
G6PD	Glucose-6-phosphate dehydrogenase	G6PD deficiency
GPI	Glucose phosphate isomerase	GPI deficiency
GSR	Glutathione reductase	GSR deficiency
HK1	Hexokinase 1	Hemolytic anemia
NT5C3	Pyrimidine 5'-nucleotidase	Hemolytic anemia
PGK1	Phosphoglycerate kinase 1	PGK1 deficiency
PKLR	Pyruvate kinase (liver and red cell)	PKLR deficiency
PKM	Pyruvate kinase (muscle)	Bloom syndrome
TPI1	Triosephosphate isomerase 1	TPI1 deficiency
GSS	Glutathione synthase	GSS deficiency
ADA	Adenosine deaminase	ADA deficiency
AK1	Adenylate kinase 1	AK1 deficiency
PFKM	Phosphofructokinase (muscle)	PFKM deficiency Glycogen storage disease type 7
PFKL	Phosphofructokinase (liver)	—
UGT1A1	UDP glycosyltransferase 1 family, polypeptide A1	Crigler-Najjar syndrome 1 and 2
UGT1A6	UDP glycosyltransferase 1 family, polypeptide A6	UGT1A6 deficiency
UGT1A7	UDP glycosyltransferase 1 family, polypeptide A7	UGT1A7 deficiency
SLCO1B1	Solute carrier organic anion transporter family, member 1B1	Rotor syndrome
SLCO1B3	Solute carrier organic anion transporter family, member 1B3	Rotor syndrome

Data from Refs.[22–24]

may want to be vigilant about this possibility as a cause of early hyperbilirubinemia. At least 1 prospective, multicenter study is underway to better assess this potential risk.

AFTER IDENTIFICATION OF HEMOLYSIS IN A JAUNDICED PRETERM INFANT, HOW IS EXACT CAUSE FOUND?

In many instances of hemolytic jaundice in a preterm neonate, the cause of the jaundice is obvious. Examples include direct antiglobulin test (DAT) or Coombs-positive ABO hemolytic jaundice, ABO incompatibility with negative DAT, heavy bruising, bacterial sepsis, internal hemorrhages, and DIC. In other instances, the underlying cause of hemolysis is obscure. Essentially all of the various causes of hemolytic jaundice among term neonates can also be the causes of hemolytic jaundice among preterm neonates.[14] Hereditary spherocytosis, pyruvate kinase deficiency, glucose-6-phosphate dehydrogenase (G6PD) deficiency, and all other hemolytic conditions caused by genetic mutations in erythrocyte membrane proteins or enzymes, should be considered when the more common causes of significant hemolytic jaundice in premature neonates have been excluded.

When initial efforts to identify the cause of ongoing hemolysis fail, next-generation sequencing (NGS) tests can be of value. Developed only a few years ago, these are currently being adopted by clinical reference laboratories as diagnostic tests for mutations or polymorphisms causing various genetically based disorders. Because multiple candidate genes from 1 patient can be sequenced in parallel in a single run, the cost of the procedure can be several orders of magnitude less than previous methods in which mutations were sought by sequencing candidate genes 1 at a time. Moreover, using a barcoding technique to identify which DNA fragments belong to which patients, the DNA of multiple patients can be sequenced in a single run, further reducing costs. The test usually reports the exact mutation and not only the gene involved.

Best practices

What is current practice?

- Premature neonates with hyperbilirubinemia, regardless of an identified hemolytic process, are managed with phototherapy, and very rarely with exchange transfusion.

- It is possible that hyperbilirubinemia associated with hemolysis is more damaging to premature neonates than to term neonates.

- It is possible that hemolytic jaundice is more damaging to premature neonates than is nonhemolytic jaundice, perhaps because the rate of TB rise can be steeper with hemolysis.

- It is possible that hemolysis and jaundice may be masked in premature neonates due to an effective or mature bilirubin clearance process as well as the visual recognition of jaundice.

What changes in current practice are likely to improve outcomes?

- Identifying hemolysis as a mechanism causing jaundice in a preterm infant can alert clinicians to the need for an earlier use of prophylactic intensive phototherapy and to the high likelihood of bilirubin rebound after the phototherapy is discontinued.

- Recognizing hemolysis as an underlying cause of hyperbilirubinemia can facilitate anticipatory guidance of these infants, throughout their hospitalization and at home, thereby avoiding adverse outcomes of hyperbilirubinemia and anemia.

- Appreciating that a fraction of donor RBCs have lysed during storage, and can lyse during or after transfusion, will alert clinicians to the possibility of a sudden and unanticipated increase in TB levels immediately following RBC transfusions of premature neonates.

When novel mutations or genetically complex conditions are present, involving mutations in several genes, NGS can identify the situation, whereas previous techniques frequently did not.

The quality of genetic data generated by NGS and the usefulness to clinical diagnosis has already generated NGS availability for diagnosing the cause of congenital hemolytic jaundice. Thus, NGS panels like the one illustrated in **Table 3** to identify the underlying genetic causes of neonatal jaundice, are available from reference laboratories.[22–26]

SUMMARY

Hemolysis, an abnormally short RBC lifespan, can be an important cause of hyperbilirubinemia in premature as well as term neonates. Hemolysis can be the result of genetic abnormalities intrinsic to RBCs or factors exogenous to normal RBCs. The latter include entities that damage RBCs, such as infectious agents, chemicals, thermal injury, or physical disruption of RBCs such as that which occurs in DIC. Hemolysis in neonates can lead to (1) a relatively rapid increase in TB, (2) hyperbilirubinemia that is somewhat slow to fall with phototherapy, or (3) hyperbilirubinemia that is likely to rebound after phototherapy is discontinued. The laboratory methods for diagnosing hemolysis in term infants are more difficult to apply, or less conclusive, in preterm infants. Transfusion of donor RBCs to preterm neonates can present a bilirubin load that must be metabolized. The load is approximately proportional to the amount of hemolysis of donor RBCs before, during, or after transfusion. The cause of hemolytic jaundice in premature infants is generally straightforward but can be obscure. Genetic causes can be identified, in cases of severe hemolytic jaundice of obscure origin, by NGS panels.

REFERENCES

1. Glader G, Allen GA. Neonatal hemolysis. In: deAlarcon PA, Werner EJ, Christensen RD, editors. Neonatal hematology. 2nd edition. Cambridge (United Kingdom): Cambridge University Press; 2014. p. 91.
2. Franco R. Measurement of red cell lifespan and aging. Transfus Med Hemother 2012;39:302–7.
3. Mock DM, Matthews NI, Zhu S, et al. Red blood cell (RBC) survival determined in humans using RBCs labeled at multiple biotin densities. Transfusion 2011;51:1047–57.
4. Pearson HA. Life-span of the fetal red blood cell. J Pediatr 1967;70:166–71.
5. Franco RS. The measurement and importance of red cell survival. Am J Hematol 2009;84:109–14.
6. Kuruvilla DJ, Nalbant D, Widness JA, et al. Mean remaining life span: a new clinically relevant parameter to assess the quality of transfused red blood cells. Transfusion 2014;54(10 Pt 2):2724–9.
7. Mock DM, Widness JA, Veng-Pedersen P, et al. Measurement of posttransfusion red cell survival with the biotin label. Transfus Med Rev 2014;28:114–25.
8. Gallagher PG. Abnormalities of the erythrocyte membrane. Pediatr Clin North Am 2013;60:1349–62.
9. Stevenson DK, Vreman HJ, Wong RJ. Bilirubin production and the risk of bilirubin neurotoxicity. Semin Perinatol 2011;35:121–6.
10. Cohen RS, Wong RJ, Stevenson DK. Understanding neonatal jaundice: a perspective on causation. Pediatr Neonatol 2010;51:143–8.

11. Maisels MJ, Pathak A, Nelson NM, et al. Endogenous production of carbon monoxide in normal and erythroblastotic newborn infants. J Clin Invest 1971;50:1–8.
12. Maisels MJ, Kring E. The contribution of hemolysis to early jaundice in normal newborns. Pediatrics 2006;118:276–9.
13. Kaplan M, Bromiker R, Hammerman C. Hyperbilirubinemia, hemolysis, and increased bilirubin neurotoxicity. Semin Perinatol 2014;38:429–37.
14. Christensen RD, Yaish HM. Hemolytic disorders causing severe neonatal hyperbilirubinemia. Clin Perinatol 2015;42:515–27.
15. Christensen RD, Lambert DK, Henry E, et al. End-tidal carbon monoxide as an indicator of the hemolytic rate. Blood Cells Mol Dis 2015;54:292–6.
16. Christensen RD, Malleske DT, Lambert DK, et al. Measuring end-tidal carbon monoxide of jaundiced neonates in the birth hospital to identify those with hemolysis. Neonatology 2015;109:1–5.
17. Christensen RD, Henry E, Andres RL, et al. Neonatal reference ranges for blood concentrations of nucleated red blood cells. Neonatology 2010;99:289–94.
18. Christensen RD, Henry E, Yaish HM, et al. Reference intervals for reticulocyte counts and reticulocyte parameters of neonates. J Perinatol 2016;36:61–6.
19. Christensen RD, Yaish HM, Lemons RS. Neonatal hemolytic jaundice: morphologic features of erythrocytes that will help you diagnose the underlying condition. Neonatology 2014;105:243–9.
20. Christensen RD, Baer VL, Snow GL, et al. Association of neonatal red blood cell transfusion with increase in serum bilirubin. Transfusion 2014;54:3068–74.
21. Ozment CP, Mamo LB, Campbell ML, et al. Transfusion-related biologic effects and free hemoglobin, heme, and iron. Transfusion 2013;53:732–40.
22. Christensen RD, Nussenzveig RH, Yaish HM, et al. Causes of hemolysis in neonates with extreme hyperbilirubinemia. J Perinatol 2014;34:616–9.
23. Yaish HM, Christensen RD, Agarwal A. A neonate with Coombs-negative hemolytic jaundice with spherocytes but normal erythrocyte indices: a rare case of autosomal-recessive hereditary spherocytosis due to alpha-spectrin deficiency. J Perinatol 2013;33:404–6.
24. Nussenzveig RH, Christensen RD, Prchal JT, et al. Novel α-spectrin mutation in trans with α-spectrin causing severe neonatal jaundice from hereditary spherocytosis. Neonatology 2014;106:355–7.
25. Maisels MJ. Screening and early postnatal management strategies to prevent hazardous hyperbilirubinemia in newborns of 35 or more weeks of gestation. Semin Fetal Neonatal Med 2010;15:129–35.
26. Hulzebos CV, van Imhoff DE, Bos AF, et al. Usefulness of the bilirubin/albumin ratio for predicting bilirubin- induced neurotoxicity in premature infants. Arch Dis Child Fetal Neonatal Ed 2008;93:F384–8.

Bilirubin Binding Capacity in the Preterm Neonate

Sanjiv B. Amin, MBBS, MD, MS

KEYWORDS

- Total serum bilirubin • Unbound bilirubin • Bilirubin:albumin molar ratio
- Bilirubin–albumin binding affinity • Bilirubin-induced neurotoxicity

KEY POINTS

- Bilirubin–albumin binding limits the use of total serum/plasma bilirubin (TB) as an indicator of bilirubin-induced neurotoxicity in premature infants.
- Bilirubin binding capacity and affinity are low and variable in premature infants.
- Specific exogenous drugs, intravenous lipids, and clinical factors such as metabolic acidosis, hypothermia, hypoxia, and sepsis may adversely affect bilirubin–albumin binding.
- The bilirubin:albumin molar ratio, in conjunction with TB, may be useful as a marker of bilirubin-induced neurotoxicity in more mature preterm and late preterm infants.
- Unbound bilirubin is a better vascular gauge of hyperbilirubinemia "severity" for bilirubin-induced neurotoxicity than the conventionally measured TB in premature infants.

INTRODUCTION

The primary goal of the evaluation and management of unconjugated hyperbilirubinemia in premature infants is to prevent acute and chronic bilirubin-induced neurotoxicity, a spectrum of neurodevelopmental disorders including, but not limited to, central apnea, sensorineural deafness, auditory neuropathy spectrum disorder, language disorders, autism, upward gaze palsy, and athetoid cerebral palsy.[1–10] It is generally believed that premature infants are at increased risk for bilirubin-induced neurotoxicity compared with term infants.[4,11] However, to date the evidence-based management of hyperbilirubinemia to prevent bilirubin-induced neurotoxicity remains elusive in premature infants less than 35 weeks gestational age (GA).[12] Consensus-based management guidelines for hyperbilirubinemia using total serum/plasma bilirubin (TB) levels, GA, and clinical risk factors for premature infants less than 35 weeks GA were recently published.[11] The TB level, the traditional parameter to

Disclosure Statement: The author has nothing to disclose.
The work was supported by NIH R21 HD078744, NIH R21 DE021161, and NIH R03HD61084.
Division of Neonatology, Department of Pediatrics, University of Rochester School of Medicine and Dentistry, Box 651, 601 Elmwood Avenue, Rochester, NY 14642, USA
E-mail address: Sanjiv_Amin@urmc.rochester.edu

Clin Perinatol 43 (2016) 241–257
http://dx.doi.org/10.1016/j.clp.2016.01.003
perinatology.theclinics.com

evaluate and manage hyperbilirubinemia in premature infants, has not been a useful predictor of acute and chronic bilirubin-induced neurotoxicity.[4,13–19] This is not surprising; several biochemical and physiologic factors are involved in the pathogenesis of bilirubin-induced neurotoxicity.[20] More specifically, bilirubin–albumin binding limits the use of TB as an indicator of the amount of bilirubin in vascular and extravascular compartments, the magnitude of ongoing bilirubin production/excretion mismatch, and the overall risk of bilirubin toxicity in premature infants. There is growing evidence that non–albumin-bound (unbound) or free bilirubin (UB), resulting from altered bilirubin–albumin binding, is a more sensitive and specific biochemical measure of acute and chronic bilirubin-induced neurotoxicity than TB. In this article, bilirubin–albumin binding, a modifying factor for bilirubin-induced neurotoxicity, in premature infants is discussed. The endogenous and exogenous factors that may influence the bilirubin–albumin binding in premature infants is also examined. Furthermore, existing evidence for the role of bilirubin:albumin molar ratio (BAMR) and UB as predictors of bilirubin-induced neurotoxicity in premature infants is provided.

Bilirubin–Albumin Biochemical Structure and Binding

The predominant native form of unconjugated bilirubin in its usual form ($4Z,15Z$-IXα isomer) has its 2 rigid dipyrrole units internally hydrogen bonded to each other such that no polar (or ionizable) groups are exposed making it quite insoluble in water at a neutral pH.[21,22] Because of its low solubility in water, free unconjugated bilirubin can form detrimental dimers and higher aggregates.[22] Solubility increases with increasing pH owing to the ionization of the acidic groups on the molecule.[21,22] The hydrophobic native form of unconjugated bilirubin can readily cross the phospholipid layers of biomembranes, including the blood–brain barrier and neuronal cell membranes.[23] This native bilirubin or free unconjugated bilirubin ($4Z,15Z$-IXα isomer) is neurotoxic.[24,25]

Fortunately, native bilirubin, primarily a product of hemoglobin (Hgb) degradation, exists in the blood mostly bound to albumin, preventing it from crossing intact blood–brain barrier. Albumin serves as a vehicle for the transport of bilirubin to the liver, where the bilirubin dissociates from albumin and enters the hepatic cell for conjugation. More important, albumin is a highly abundant serum protein (0.6 mmol/L), which comprises 50% to 60% of the total plasma protein in humans. Moreover, albumin is a 66-kDa monomer containing 3 homologous helical domains (I–III), each divided into A and B subdomains.[26] It is therefore not surprising that, in addition to bilirubin, albumin binds a wide variety of endogenous ligands, including nonesterified fatty acids and hemin, all of them acidic and lipophilic compounds, with high affinity at multiple sites.[27–29] Among exogenous substances, many commonly used drugs with acidic or electronegative features (eg, ibuprofen) also bind to human serum albumin, usually at 1 of 2 primary sites located in subdomains IIA and IIIA.[27]

There are at least 2 types of binding sites for bilirubin and its photoisomers on albumin.[30,31] The strongest and key binding site for native bilirubin has a very high binding constant (affinity), approximately 1.4×10^7 L/mol at 37°C, and can be considered a specific site.[32,33] Other secondary sites have at least a 10-fold lower binding affinity.[34] Recent studies indicate that there are site-to-site interactions or allosteric interaction within albumin.[35–37] It is known that fatty acid and drug binding to albumin induces conformational changes in albumin, which may then influence bilirubin–albumin binding.[29,35–37]

Bilirubin–Albumin Binding Capacity and Affinity

Bilirubin–albumin binding is a function of the concentrations of bilirubin and albumin, and the binding affinity for bilirubin (strength of bilirubin binding to albumin).

The fraction of UB increases significantly as the TB approaches the binding capacity of albumin (1 g human serum albumin binds approximately 8 mg of bilirubin in term infants and much less in premature infants) or when the apparent binding affinity decreases.

Because of the large quantity of albumin and its' very high affinity for bilirubin, the serum UB level is essentially controlled by the bilirubin binding capacity (BBC) in healthy late preterm and term neonates.[33,38] Binding capacity is generally defined as the concentration of the bound ligand at infinite ligand concentrations.[39] For BBC at a high-affinity binding site, consideration has to be given to the following equilibrium:

Albumin (R) + Unbound Bilirubin (UB) $\rightleftarrows$ Albumin Bound Bilirubin (B)

Where R represents the concentration of albumin with an empty high-affinity site or the reserve albumin binding capacity and B represents the concentration of albumin with bilirubin bound to a high-affinity site. The total BBC is the total amount of albumin capable of strongly binding bilirubin (R + B) at the high-affinity site. The relationship assumes that the binding protein, albumin, has specific, noninteractive, and independent binding sites.[34,40] The relationship does not account for bilirubin binding to low-affinity sites and other proteins or possible bilirubin displacement by competitors. Furthermore, allosteric interaction, aforementioned, may alter the total BBC in premature infants. In addition, problems with bilirubin aggregation and solubility as UB increases make it impossible to obtain complete binding isotherms (ie, binding isotherms in which the albumin-bound bilirubin reaches a level that changes little with additional increases in TB).[40,41] Several methods have been used to measure total and reserve BBC and provide indirect estimation of UB; however, each method is associated with some limitations.[42] It may be more helpful to consider the albumin concentration (or BAMR) as a practical "BBC," whereas newer and better technology to measure BBC in premature infants is being developed and validated for research and clinical use.[42]

It is also important to recognize that bilirubin–albumin binding is reversible and that there is a dynamic equilibrium with bilirubin binding onto albumin and dissociating off continuously at normal serum pH and temperature.[43] As bilirubin leaves the blood compartment and enters the tissues, more bilirubin is dissociating from the albumin-bound pool. The bilirubin exits into the tissues at a rate that is, proportional to the UB concentration. Thus, serum UB, TB, and albumin concentrations are related by the law of mass action and characterized by an affinity or binding constant, K, as shown in the equation below:

$$\frac{TB - UB}{K([Albumin] - TB + UB)} = UB$$

The law of mass equation indicates that the UB is inversely proportional to albumin and its intrinsic ability to bind bilirubin (K). The relationship clearly explains the influence of bilirubin–albumin binding (BBC and affinity) on UB and the risk for bilirubin-induced neurotoxicity. The relationship also underscores the importance of evaluating bilirubin–albumin binding in addition to TB to indirectly determine the risk for bilirubin-induced neurotoxicity.

If a UB level is available, the bilirubin-binding constant (K), a measure of the strength of the binding or binding affinity, can be calculated using the mass equation as:

$$\frac{TB - UB}{UB([Albumin] - TB + UB)} = K$$

Bilirubin–Albumin Binding as a Function of Gestational Age and Postnatal Age

Few data are available on the ontogeny of BBC and affinity in premature infants. There is general agreement that serum albumin levels and BBC is lower in premature compared with term infants.[11,12,44,45] Bender and colleagues[46] using the fifth-day blood sample demonstrated that BBC at a high-affinity site improves with increasing GA in infants less than 31 weeks GA. However, the findings were based on a single peroxidase concentration and several tenuous assumptions of bilirubin–albumin binding.[40] Similarly, Lamola and colleagues[47] showed a positive correlation ($r = 0.53$) between GA and BBC measured by 2 different versions of the hematofluorometric instrument in 3 different cohorts of premature and term infants. They reported an increase in BBC by 1 mg/dL per week with increasing GA.[47] Interestingly, there was no association of BBC with sepsis in their cohort.[47] The hematofluorometric instrument assumes a single, noninteractive, high-affinity binding site on albumin.[42] Cashore and colleagues[48] using the Sephadex method reported that BBC remains unchanged during the first 10 days of life in healthy preterm and term infants; however, BBC is highly variable in sick infants.

In a large, prospective study using the modified peroxidase method, Amin and colleagues[49] reported that in more mature preterm infants (>30 weeks GA), the binding affinity improves over the first week, whereas in infants less than 30 weeks GA, bilirubin-binding affinity varies within and between infants, but overall, decreases during the first postnatal week. This variability in bilirubin binding affinity in premature infants has been reported previously using the Sephadex method.[45] Several exogenous and endogenous factors described elsewhere in this paper may contribute to this variability in bilirubin binding affinity in premature infants.

Clinical Risk Factors and Bilirubin–Albumin Binding

Various clinical factors such as hypothermia, hypoxia, acidosis, asphyxia, and sepsis have been postulated to explain the occurrence of bilirubin-induced neurotoxicity at much lower TB levels in premature infants.[4,12] These factors are thought to increase the risk of bilirubin-induced neurotoxicity by not only affecting the bilirubin–albumin binding, but also by facilitating bilirubin entry into the brain, and/or neuronal uptake of bilirubin.[4] In an earlier study involving 76 infants, reserve albumin concentration determined by dialysis with ^{14}C-monoacetyl diamino diphenyl sulfone was decreased and the bilirubin toxicity index was increased in the presence of clinical risk factors (hypoxia, acidosis, or sepsis), suggesting an increased risk of bilirubin-induced neurotoxicity in the presence of these risk factors.[50] Meisel and colleagues[51] evaluated the influence of acid–base status on bilirubin–albumin binding in 254 low birthweight (LBW) infants at the ages of 3, 4, 5, and 8 days and reported a weak, but significant, correlation between metabolic acidosis and the bilirubin:reserve albumin ratio as well as the bilirubin toxicity index. A decrease in bilirubin–albumin binding and a doubling of the toxic potential of bilirubin occurred with shifts to a metabolically acidic state with a base deficit of 10.[51] In another study, involving 11 late preterm infants, the correction of a metabolic acidosis (pH 7.12–7.34) during the first postnatal day resulted in an improvement of apparent bilirubin–albumin binding affinity and a decrease in UB levels.[52] Although the exact mechanism is unclear, neonatal sepsis by decreasing albumin production and increasing free fatty acid (FFA) concentration, a known bilirubin displacer, may adversely influence bilirubin–albumin binding.[53,54] Ritter and colleagues[55] reported in a small prospective study involving premature infants that prolonged hypoxia (Pao$_2$ <50 mm Hg), prolonged acidosis (pH <7.1) and prolonged hypothermia (<35.5°C) occurring before peak UB levels were significant clinical risk factors for kernicterus. Both hypoxia and hypothermia may also increase concentrations of FFA, known bilirubin displacers. Although Kim and colleagues[56] failed to identify a single or combination of risk factors to be useful in predicting the development of kernicterus in premature infants, the incidence of severe acidosis and hypoxic encephalopathy was higher in infants with kernicterus (n = 27) compared with normal infants (n = 103). Compared with these studies, Turkel and colleagues[57] in a small retrospective matched control study of 64 infants, failed to identify any clinical risk factor associated with kernicterus in premature infants. Clearly, the role of these clinical risk factors in the pathogenesis of bilirubin-induced neurotoxicity needs to be evaluated further in premature infants. In the meantime, the weak evidence derived from observational studies warrants a more aggressive management of hyperbilirubinemia in the presence of 1 or more clinical risk factors as also recently recommended by the expert committee.[12]

Phototherapy and Bilirubin–Albumin Binding

Phototherapy is the mainstay of therapy in premature infants. In jaundiced newborns, bilirubin photoisomers, mainly *4Z,15E*-bilirubin and *Z*-lumirubin, comprise approximately 10% of TB before phototherapy, and increase to as much as approximately 30% during phototherapy.[58–60] Earlier in vitro studies reported that the photoisomers bind much less avidly to plasma proteins than to native *4Z,15Z*-bilirubin, and UB levels should therefore increase during phototherapy.[61,62] However, the issue regarding neurotoxic properties of photoisomers remains as an unresolved issue.[63] If *4Z,15E*-bilirubin is not neurotoxic, UB measured by the peroxidase method may overestimate the toxic UB fraction by up to 30%.[58,59,63] However, if it is neurotoxic, UB remains an "accurate" measure of toxic bilirubin isomers, even during phototherapy. The available, but limited, literature also suggests that the peroxidase test commonly used to measure UB seems to be more specific for native *4Z,15Z*-bilirubin than the photoisomers produced by phototherapy.[62,64] Although a recent in vitro study reported a disproportionate decrease in UB relative to the decrease in the concentration of *4Z,15Z*-bilirubin, the clinical studies performed thus far suggest little change with phototherapy in bilirubin–albumin binding as assessed by the peroxidase test.[58,65–67] This interaction with photoisomers will need to be investigated with any newer assays of bilirubin–albumin binding that may be developed and used in the future.[42]

Exogenous Drugs and Bilirubin–Albumin Binding

Several therapeutic drugs and preservatives used in preparing these drugs have been studied and shown in in vitro studies to displace bilirubin from albumin binding sites with different levels of activity (**Table 1**).[68–72] Of the drugs studied, the most potent bilirubin displacers are sulfamethoxazole, sulfisoxazole, sulfadiazine, and ceftriaxone. The potential for abnormal binding may persist for the first 10 to 12 weeks in premature infants.[39] Therefore, drugs with a strong bilirubin displacing effect should be avoided as long as there is a risk for bilirubin-induced neurotoxicity in premature infants. Also, any new drugs with acidic or electronegative features and high protein binding should be evaluated for a bilirubin displacing effect before routine clinical use in neonates, as was considered for ibuprofen use in premature infants.

Several in vitro studies performed using bilirubin–albumin solution or pooled newborn sera have shown that the risk of a ibuprofen-induced bilirubin displacing effect depends on the plasma concentration of ibuprofen, BAMR, and the intrinsic ability of albumin to bind ibuprofen and bilirubin.[73–75] Ahlfors and colleagues[74] demonstrated, using the peroxidase method, that a significant increase in UB concentration

Table 1
Drugs and bilirubin displacing effect

Drugs with Moderate to Strong Displacing Effect	Drugs with Minimal Displacing Effect	Drugs with No Displacing Effect
Sulfamethoxazole	Nafcillin	Aminoglycosides
Sulfisoxazole	Ampicillin	Insulin
Sulfadiazine	Oxacillin	Dopamine
Ceftriaxone	Methicillin	Dobutamine
Cefotetan	Furosemide	Morphine
Moxalactam	Phenobarbital	Fentanyl
Dicloxacillin	Papavarine	Indomethacin
Carbenicillin	Caffeine	Vitamins
Cefazolin	Aminophylline	Diazepam
Ibuprofen	Cefotaxime	Thyroxine

was only observed at ibuprofen concentrations greater than 50 μg/mL in 2 pooled newborn sera with BAMRs of 0.3 and 0.36. Similarly, Cooper-Peel and colleagues[75] demonstrated that, with a reverse displacement method using cord sera with a BAMR of 0.5, there was no to minimal bilirubin displacing effect with ibuprofen concentrations less than 50 μg/mL. However, there was an increase in UB by a factor of 4 with an ibuprofen concentration of 154 μg/mL (750 μmol/L). Compared with in vitro studies, Amin and Miravalle,[76] using the modified peroxidase method, reported that intravenous ibuprofen, when used at the recommended dosage for the management of patent ductus arteriosus after the first 2 postnatal days, is not associated with a bilirubin displacing effect in relatively stable premature infants (<30 weeks GA) with a BAMR of less than 0.5. This finding was confirmed subsequently by Desfrere and colleagues[77] in stable premature infants (<32 weeks GA) with mild to moderate hyperbilirubinemia and a BAMR of less than 0.3.

The accumulated evidence from clinical studies in premature infants suggests that clinically significant displacement is unlikely if intravenous ibuprofen is used with the recommended dosage after the first 2 postnatal days and with a BAMR of less than 0.5. However, until further data are available, caution is warranted in using intravenous ibuprofen in infants with a BAMR of greater than 0.5 and during the first 2 postnatal days, when the plasma levels of ibuprofen may be higher.[78]

Intralipid and Bilirubin–Albumin Binding

The clearance of FFA is slower in premature than in term infants, and intralipid (IL) intake in premature infants may result in elevated FFA levels.[79–81] FFA bind to albumin at 3 sites. The first 2 mol of FFA preferentially bind to its first 2 binding sites. The third binding site of FFA to albumin is also the high affinity site of bilirubin to albumin. When the FFA:albumin molar ratio is 4:1 or greater, FFA compete with bilirubin at the primary site of bilirubin (also the third binding site of FFA) resulting in displacement of bilirubin.[82] Earlier studies that demonstrated the adverse effects of IL on bilirubin–albumin binding were based on indirect estimation of UB or using a single peroxide concentration in more mature infants.[34,79,82–91] The effect of a gradual increase in IL (20%) intake from 1.5 to 3.0 g/kg per day during the first postnatal week on bilirubin–albumin binding, as measured by the modified peroxidase test using an UB analyzer, was evaluated in 62, 24 to 33 weeks GA infants.[92] At each IL dose greater than 1.5 g/kg per day, there was statistically significant lower binding affinity in infants

28 weeks or less GA (n = 32) compared with infants greater than 2 weeks GA (n = 30). There were also significantly higher UB concentrations, despite significantly lower TB concentrations, at each IL dose 1.5 g/kg per day or greater in 28 weeks or less GA infants compared with infants greater than 28 weeks GA. The cumulative frequency of elevated UB concentrations (>1 μg/dL or >17.1 nmol/L, a level that may be associated with neurotoxicity in premature infants) as a function of IL intake was inversely related to GA and was significantly different between 2-week GA groups: 24 to 26, $26^{1/7}$ to 28, $28^{1/7}$ to 30, and $30^{1/7}$ to 32 weeks GA infants (**Table 2**). The amount of IL intake that is tolerated without decreasing bilirubin binding affinity and secondary increase in UB increases with GA. An IL intake of 1.5 or greater and 2.0 g/kg per day was associated with UB concentrations greater than 1 μg/dL in 24 to 26 and $26^{1/7}$ to 28 weeks GA infants, respectively.

The causal relationship between IL intake and bilirubin–albumin binding variables as measured by the modified peroxidase method was subsequently evaluated in 24 to 33 weeks GA infants.[93] In 28 weeks or less GA infants, there was a statistically significant association between IL intake and FFA or FFA:albumin molar ratio. The FFA:albumin molar ratio also predicted bilirubin–albumin binding affinity. As the FFA:albumin molar ratio increased with increasing IL intake, bilirubin–albumin binding affinity decreased. Binding affinity predicted UB, and a decrease in binding affinity correlated significantly with an increase in UB. However, in infants greater than 28 weeks GA, IL intake was not associated significantly with FFA concentrations or FFA:albumin molar ratios. Therefore, FFA or FFA:albumin molar ratio is not a mediator of any increase in UB with IL intake in infants greater than 28 weeks GA. These findings provide an explanation for why higher IL intake may not be associated with an increase in UB concentrations in infants greater than 28 weeks GA. The available evidence suggests that IL intake should be appropriately limited in infants 28 weeks or less GA during the first postnatal week when unconjugated hyperbilirubinemia is common.[90,92,93]

Bilirubin:Albumin Molar Ratio and Risk for Bilirubin-Induced Neurotoxicity

The consensus-based guidelines for the management of hyperbilirubinemia recommends measurement of serum albumin in premature infants.[11] Scheidt and colleagues[18] reported the neurodevelopmental outcomes at 6 years in 224 infants less than 2000 g who participated in the National Institute of Child Health and Development Neonatal Research Network randomized phototherapy trial. There was no association of TB or BAMR with neurodevelopmental outcomes, including cerebral palsy and

Table 2
Incidence of EUB concentration (>1 μg/dL) as a function of IL intake in 24–33 weeks GA infants

	24–26 wk GA (n = 11)	$26^{1/7}$–28 wk GA (n = 21)	$28^{1/7}$–30 wk GA (n = 11)	$30^{1/7}$–32 wk GA (n = 11)	$32^{1/7}$–33 wk GA (n = 8)	P
n (%) subjects with EUB @ IL 1.5 g/kg/d	4 (36)	1 (5)	0 (0)	0 (0)	0 (0)	.015
n (%) subjects with EUB @ IL 2 g/kg/d	5 (45)	5 (24)	0 (0)	0 (0)	0 (0)	.009
n (%) subjects with EUB @ IL 2.5 g/kg/d	6 (55)	7 (33)	0 (0)	0 (0)	0 (0)	.001
n (%) subjects with EUB @ IL 3 g/kg/d	5(63)	10 (77)	0 (0)	0 (0)	0 (0)	<.001

Abbreviations: EUB, elevated unbound bilirubin; GA, gestational age; IL, intravenous lipid.

intellectual disability, after controlling for neonatal risk factors.[18] Similarly, Cashore and Oh,[94] in a small retrospective study, reported no significant difference in TB, albumin, or BAMR between 5 premature infants (mean GA, 29.2 weeks) with autopsy-proven kernicterus compared with 8 premature infants (mean GA, 28.1 weeks) without kernicterus.

However, several others have reported on the possible role of albumin or BAMR in premature infants. Kim and colleagues[56] in a retrospective matched control study involving premature and term infants (24–42 weeks GA) reported no differences in peak TB between 27 infants (mean GA, 32 weeks) with autopsy findings of kernicterus and 103 control infants (mean GA, 31 weeks) without kernicterus. In a subset of the study population, the mean serum albumin concentration (2.0 ± 0.8 g/dL) in the 14 infants with kernicterus was significantly lower compared with the 33 control infants (2.6 ± 0.5 g/dL), indicating that peak BAMR was higher in infants with kernicterus compared with control infants.[56] Ritter and colleagues[55] also reported no significant difference in peak TB and albumin levels between 7 premature infants (mean GA, 28.3 weeks) with autopsy-proven kernicterus and 23 premature infants (mean GA, 28.5 weeks) without kernicterus; however, calculated peak BAMRs were higher in infants with kernicterus compared with those without kernicterus (0.29 vs 0.25). Amin and colleagues[95] using sequential auditory brainstem evoked response (ABR) during the first 2 postnatal weeks, compared TB and BAMRs as predictors of acute bilirubin encephalopathy, as defined by abnormal ABR maturational changes in 143 infants who were delivered as 28 to 32 weeks GA. There was no difference ($P = .98$) in mean peak TB between infants with normal ABR maturation and abnormal ABR maturation. Although BAMRs did not predict abnormal ABR maturation, the trend ($P = .19$) was better than that for TB. In a subset of 45 premature infants, in whom UB was measured, peak BAMR, but not peak TB, was significantly higher in infants with abnormal ABR maturation compared with infants with normal ABR maturation.[95] In a recent study involving late preterm and term infants with severe hyperbilirubinemia in Egypt, both TB and BAMR were significantly associated with bilirubin-induced neurotoxicity; however, BAMR failed to provide any advantage over TB for predicting bilirubin-induced neurotoxicity.[96] A recent multicenter randomized trial in the Netherlands studied the usefulness of BAMR combined with TB compared with TB alone in the management of hyperbilirubinemia and reported no additional benefit of using BAMR in the management of hyperbilirubinemia in infants 32 weeks or less GA. However, in a subgroup analysis of infants with greater than 1000 g, the use of BAMR, in addition to TB, was associated with reduction in mortality compared with TB alone.[97] Furthermore, a recent case series of 5 sick premature infants who developed MRI findings of kernicterus with peak TB concentrations ranging from 8.7 to 11.9 mg/dL and serum albumin concentrations ranging from 1.4 to 2.1 g/dL (BAMR >0.47) underscores the importance of measurement of serum albumin in premature infants.[98]

The existing evidence suggests that BAMR is better than TB as a predictor of bilirubin-induced neurotoxicity in premature infants, and serum albumin should be routinely measured and used for the management of hyperbilirubinemia in premature infants. Future prospective bilirubin toxicity studies in premature infants should continue to evaluate the usefulness of BAMR as a function of GA.

Bilirubin–Albumin Binding and Neurodevelopmental Outcomes in Premature Infants

The findings of earlier studies correlating bilirubin–albumin binding test results with poor neurologic outcomes were very promising.[99–103] A highly significant association of low reserve BBC with abnormal communication skills and language functions at 7 years of age after controlling for known confounders was reported in 30 to 41 weeks GA infants with moderate to severe hyperbilirubinemia.[10] These earlier studies of bilirubin–albumin binding status and neurodevelopmental outcomes involved binding tests such as the Sephadex gel filtration method for BBC, dye binding method for reserve BBC, and salicylate saturation index for bilirubin binding affinity.[42] Despite encouraging results, these bilirubin–albumin binding tests failed to find clinical application, most likely owing to the disappearance of kernicterus around the same time period. However, several factors including the development of the peroxidase method to measure UB, reappearance of kernicterus in developed countries with early newborn discharge, acknowledgment of the high prevalence of kernicterus in the developing world, and identification of ABR as a valid objective assessment tool to evaluate bilirubin toxicity during the neonatal period in premature infants renewed interest in the field.[42,95,104]

Cashore and Oh[94] reported a significantly lower BBC, lower bilirubin binding affinity, and higher UB levels measured using the peroxidase method on 5 premature infants with autopsy-proven kernicterus compared with 8 premature infants without kernicterus. In the same year, Ritter and colleagues[55] reported higher UB concentrations in 7 infants with kernicterus compared with 23 infants without kernicterus in a prospective study. Since then, several studies have evaluated the usefulness of UB as a predictor of bilirubin-induced neurotoxicity in premature infants.[2,3,95,105,106] Nakamura and colleagues[105] in a prospective study compared peak TB and peak UB in LBW infants as predictors of kernicterus, which was defined as one of the following: signs of acute bilirubin encephalopathy, autopsy findings of kernicterus, infants surviving with choreoathetosis, spastic paresis, and sensorineural hearing loss. Both peak TB and peak UB levels were higher in 5 very LBW (<1500 g) infants with kernicterus compared with 45 very LBW infants without kernicterus. Similarly, both peak TB and peak UB levels were significantly higher in 7 LBW (1500–2499 g) infants with kernicterus compared with 81 LBW infants without kernicterus. However, on comparing receiver operator characteristic curves, the sensitivity and specificity of UB was better than TB in both the groups. In the very LBW group, the sensitivity and specificity for kernicterus was 100% and 96%, respectively, for a UB level of 0.8 μg/dL. In the LBW group, the sensitivity and specificity for kernicterus was 100% and 98%, respectively, for a UB level of 1.0 μg/dL.

More recent studies have used the ABR to evaluate bilirubin–albumin binding variables in premature infants. Amin and colleagues[95] in a prospective study involving 28 to 32 weeks GA infants reported that peak UB, but not peak TB, was significantly higher in 25 infants with abnormal ABR maturation compared with 20 infants with normal ABR maturation. Furthermore, and more important, premature infants with abnormal ABR maturation had more concurrent apnea and bradycardia and required more prolonged respiratory support and methylxanthine therapy.[3] Apnea was more closely associated with serum UB levels than TB.[3] The later association has been recently reconfirmed in a prospective study involving 100 premature infants (27–33 weeks GA).[2] Premature infants were divided into 2 groups based on the median UB concentration of 0.92 μg/dL (15.73 nmol/L) in this subject population. Although there was no difference in peak TB between the 2 groups, the high UB group (mean UB, 2.3 μg/dL) had a significantly higher frequency of central apnea during the first 2 postnatal weeks compared with the low UB group (mean UB, 0.64 μg/dL) with the adjusted incidence rate ratio of 1.9 (95% confidence interval [CI], 1.2–3.2). Ahlfors and colleagues[106] in a retrospective study involving 97 infants less than 35 weeks GA reported that UB (odds ratio, 2.25; 95% CI, 1.07–4.72) and not TB (odds ratio, 0.98; 95% CI, 0.84–1.15) was strongly associated with abnormal automated ABR screening tests performed before discharge. Using receiver operator characteristic curves, both Amin and colleagues[95] and Ahlfors and colleagues[106] independently reported that UB is a more specific and sensitive predictor of bilirubin-induced neurotoxicity than TB in premature infants (**Fig. 1**A, B). Ahlfors and colleagues[106] also reported that the sensitivity and specificity of the UB:TB ratio was better compared with UB, suggesting that the risk of bilirubin-induced neurotoxicity may not be a function of UB alone, but a combination of both UB and TB, which determines the miscible pool of bilirubin and the tendency to enter tissues. In a recent study involving late preterm and term infants with severe hyperbilirubinemia, peak UB, but not peak TB, was shown to be

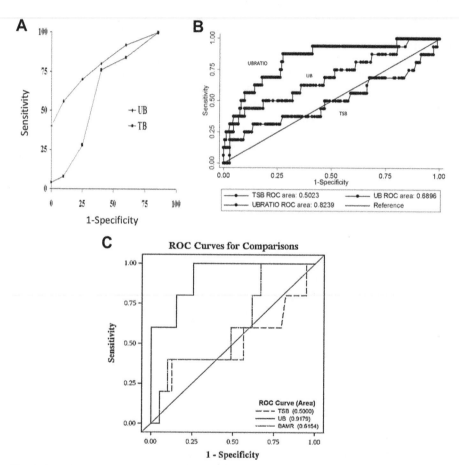

Fig. 1. Receiver operating characteristics (ROC) curves of total serum bilirubin (TB) and unbound bilirubin (UB) in premature infants as predictors of abnormal auditory brainstem evoked response maturation during the first week (*A*); ROC curves of total serum bilirubin (TSB), UB, and unbound bilirubin to total serum bilirubin ratio (UBRATIO) as predictors of an abnormal automated auditory brainstem evoked response at discharge in premature and term infants (*B*); and ROC curves of total serum bilirubin (TSB), bilirubin albumin molar ratio (BAMR) and UB as predictors of auditory dys-synchrony in late preterm and term infants (*C*). The straight line *B* and *C* is the expected curve (unity) if the variable has no predictive value (area under unity curve = 0.5). The areas under the unbound bilirubin or unbound to total serum bilirubin are significantly greater than that under the total serum bilirubin and bilirubin albumin molar ratio curves. (*From* [*A*] Amin SB, Ahlfors C, Orlando MS, et al. Bilirubin and serial auditory brainstem responses in premature infants. Pediatrics 2001;107:664–70; and [*B*] Ahlfors CE, Amin SB, Parker AE. Unbound bilirubin predicts abnormal automated auditory brainstem response in a diverse newborn population. J Perinatol 2009;29:308; with permission.)

Table 3
Unbound bilirubin and neurodevelopmental outcomes in premature infants

| | | Mean Unbound Bilirubin (μg/dL)[a] | | |
Study	GA or Birthweight (n)	No KI or Normal ABR	ABR Changes	Overt KI
Ritter et al,[55] 1982	26–32 wk GA (30)	0.65 ± 0.05	Not done	1.10 ± 0.26
Cashore & Oh,[94] 1982	≤1500 g (13)	0.76 ± 0.58	Not done	1.60 ± 0.52
Nakamura et al,[105] 1992	1500–2499 g (88)	0.54 ± 0.2	Not done	1.30 ± 0.24
	<1500 g (50)	0.46 ± 0.17		1.13 ± 0.34
Amin et al,[95] 2001	28–32 wk GA (45)	0.40 ± 0.15	0.62 ± 0.2	None
Ahlfors et al,[106] 2009	24–41 wk GA (191)	0.93 ± 0.70	1.76 ± 1.31	None
Amin,[107] 2016	≥34 wk GA with severe hyperbilirubinemia (44)	1.7 ± 0.8	4.2 ± 1.7	None

Abbreviations: ABR, auditory brainstem-evoked response; GA, gestational age; KI, kernicterus.
[a] Mean ± standard deviation.

associated with bilirubin-induced auditory dyssynchrony, a more significant and persistent neurologic outcome (**Fig. 1**C, **Table 3**).[107]

Although a well-designed, longitudinal study of the association of UB with long-term neurologic outcomes is lacking, an increasing serum UB level measured once at approximately 5 days of age using the peroxidase method in extremely LBW infants was associated with a higher risk of death or adverse neurodevelopmental outcomes regardless of clinical status.[108] Overall, these early outcome studies in premature infants provide ample evidence that UB, as measured by the peroxidase method using the UB analyzer, is associated with bilirubin-induced neurotoxicity (see **Table 3**). Second, these early outcome studies in premature infants suggest that a UB concentration of greater than 1 μg/dL measured by the modified peroxidase method using the UB analyzer may be associated with bilirubin-induced neurotoxicity in very premature infants (≤34 weeks GA). However, longitudinal studies are urgently needed to establish the critical level of UB that may be associated with acute and/or chronic bilirubin-induced neurotoxicity in premature infants.

SUMMARY

Both exogenous and endogenous factors, including certain clinical factors such as metabolic acidosis, hypoxia, sepsis, hypoalbuminemia, and hypothermia that adversely influence bilirubin–albumin binding, explains the variability in bilirubin–albumin binding in premature infants. The variability in bilirubin–albumin binding limits the usefulness of TB as a biochemical marker of bilirubin-induced neurotoxicity in premature infants. Owing to lack of valid measures to evaluate other risk factors for bilirubin-induced neurotoxicity, such as genetic susceptibility, neuronal susceptibility, and blood–brain barrier integrity, direct measurement of UB by the modified peroxidase method provides the best risk assessment of bilirubin-induced neurotoxicity for premature infants. In the most recent clinical studies that demonstrated significant association between UB and neurologic outcomes in term and premature infants, UB analyzer, a semiautomated instrument approved by the US Food and Drug Administration, was used to measure UB by the modified peroxidase method. Therefore, any newer technologies of direct and indirect measurement of UB will be required to be standardized and validated against the gold standard, modified peroxidase method using the UB analyzer before use in neonatal outcome studies.[42] Until the availability of newer assays of bilirubin–albumin binding for clinical use, the BAMR in addition to TB with consideration to known clinical risk factors, may be used as a reasonable substitute for the management of hyperbilirubinemia in premature infants.

Best practices

What is the current practice?

- TB is primarily used to evaluate and manage 34 weeks or less GA infants with unconjugated hyperbilirubinemia.

Recommendations

- Clinicians should routinely consider assessment of clinical risk factors such as hypoxia, acidosis (including perinatal asphyxia), sepsis, and hypothermia in the clinical algorithm for the management of hyperbilirubinemia.

- Albumin levels should be routinely measured in 34 weeks or less GA infants with unconjugated hyperbilirubinemia.

- In the presence of hypoalbuminemia (low BBC) and/or presence of known clinical risk factors (such as hypoxia, acidosis, etc) that may negatively influence binding affinity, treatment (phototherapy and exchange transfusion) should be considered at a much lower TB level than otherwise used in the absence of these factors.

- Hypoxia, acidosis, sepsis, and hypothermia should be prevented and/or treated aggressively in premature infants with unconjugated hyperbilirubinemia.

- As discussed in the article and shown in **Table 2**, IL intake should be appropriately limited during the first postnatal week in 28 weeks or less GA infants to decrease the incidence of elevated UB and secondary risk of bilirubin-induced neurotoxicity.

REFERENCES

1. Amin SB, Bhutani VK, Watchko JF. Apnea in acute bilirubin encephalopathy. Semin Perinatol 2014;38:407–11.
2. Amin SB, Wang H. Unbound unconjugated hyperbilirubinemia is associated with central apnea in premature infants. J Pediatr 2015;166:571–5.
3. Amin SB, Charafeddine L, Guillet R. Transient bilirubin encephalopathy and apnea of prematurity in 28 to 32 weeks gestational age infants. J Perinatol 2005;25:386–90.
4. Amin SB. Clinical assessment of bilirubin-induced neurotoxicity in premature infants. Semin Perinatol 2004;28:340–7.
5. Saluja S, Agarwal A, Kler N, et al. Auditory neuropathy spectrum disorder in late preterm and term infants with severe jaundice. Int J Pediatr Otorhinolaryngol 2010;74:1292–7.
6. Amin SB, Prinzing D, Myers G. Hyperbilirubinemia and language delay in premature infants. Pediatrics 2009;123:327–31.
7. Amin S, Smith T, Wang H. Is neonatal jaundice associated with autism spectrum disorders: a systematic review. J Autism Dev Disord 2011;41:1455–63.
8. Amin SB, Orlando M, Monczynski C, et al. Central auditory processing disorder profile in premature and term infants. Am J Perinatol 2015;32:399–404.
9. Connolly AM, Volpe JJ. Clinical features of bilirubin encephalopathy. Clin Perinatol 1990;17:371–9.
10. Johnson L, Bhutani VK. The clinical syndrome of bilirubin-induced neurologic dysfunction. Semin Perinatol 2011;35:101–13.

11. Maisels MJ, Watchko JF, Bhutani VK, et al. An approach to the management of hyperbilirubinemia in the preterm infant less than 35 weeks of gestation. J Perinatol 2012;32:660–4.

12. American Academy of Pediatrics Subcommittee on Hyperbilirubinemia. Management of hyperbilirubinemia in the newborn infant 35 or more weeks of gestation. Pediatrics 2004;114:297–316.

13. O'Shea TM, Dillard RG, Klinepeter KL, et al. Serum bilirubin levels, intracranial hemorrhage, and the risk of developmental problems in very low birth weight neonates. Pediatrics 1992;90:888–92.

14. Graziani LJ, Mitchell DG, Kornhauser M, et al. Neurodevelopment of preterm infants: neonatal neurosonographic and serum bilirubin studies. Pediatrics 1992;89:229–34.

15. van de Bor M, Ens-Dokkum M, Schreuder AM, et al. Hyperbilirubinemia in low birth weight infants and outcome at 5 years of age. Pediatrics 1992;89:359–64.

16. Ip S, Chung M, Kulig J, et al. An evidence-based review of important issues concerning neonatal hyperbilirubinemia. Pediatrics 2004;114:e130–53.

17. Newman TB, Klebanoff MA. Neonatal hyperbilirubinemia and long-term outcome: another look at the Collaborative Perinatal Project. Pediatrics 1993; 92:651–7.

18. Scheidt PC, Graubard BI, Nelson KB, et al. Intelligence at six years in relation to neonatal bilirubin levels: follow-up of the National Institute of Child Health and Human Development Clinical Trial of Phototherapy. Pediatrics 1991;87:797–805.

19. Oh W, Tyson JE, Fanaroff AA, et al. Association between peak serum bilirubin and neurodevelopmental outcomes in extremely low birth weight infants. Pediatrics 2003;112:773–9.

20. Wennberg RP, Ahlfors CE, Bhutani VK, et al. Toward understanding kernicterus: a challenge to improve the management of jaundiced newborns. Pediatrics 2006;117:474–85.

21. Ostrow JD, Mukerjee P, Tiribelli C. Structure and binding of unconjugated bilirubin: relevance for physiological and pathophysiological function. J Lipid Res 1994;35:1715–37.

22. Brodersen R. Bilirubin. Solubility and interaction with albumin and phospholipid. J Biol Chem 1979;254:2364–9.

23. Bratlid D. How bilirubin gets into the brain. Clin Perinatol 1990;17:449–65.

24. Brites D. The evolving landscape of neurotoxicity by unconjugated bilirubin: role of glial cells and inflammation. Front Pharmacol 2012;3:88.

25. Calligaris SD, Bellarosa C, Giraudi P, et al. Cytotoxicity is predicted by unbound and not total bilirubin concentration. Pediatr Res 2007;62:576–80.

26. He XM, Carter DC. Atomic structure and chemistry of human serum albumin. Nature 1992;358:209–15.

27. Peters T. All about albumin: biochemistry, genetics, and medical applications. San Diego (CA): Academic Press; 1995.

28. Sudlow G, Birkett DJ, Wade DN. The characterization of two specific drug binding sites on human serum albumin. Mol Pharmacol 1975;11:824–32.

29. Zunszain PA, Ghuman J, Komatsu T, et al. Crystal structural analysis of human serum albumin complexed with hemin and fatty acid. BMC Struct Biol 2003;3:6.

30. Goncharova I, Orlov S, Urbanova M. The location of the high- and low-affinity bilirubin-binding sites on serum albumin: ligand-competition analysis investigated by circular dichroism. Biophys Chem 2013;180-181:55–65.

31. Tran CD, Beddard GS. Interactions between bilirubin and albumins using pico-second fluorescence and circularly polarized luminescence spectroscopy. J Am Chem Soc 1982;104:6741–7.

32. Jacobsen J. Binding of bilirubin to human serum albumin - determination of the dissociation constants. FEBS Lett 1969;5:112–4.

33. Wells R, Hammond K, Lamola AA, et al. Relationships of bilirubin binding parameters. Clin Chem 1982;28:432–9.

34. Brodersen R. Binding of bilirubin to albumin. CRC Crit Rev Clin Lab Sci 1980;11: 305–99.

35. Huang BX, Dass C, Kim HY. Probing conformational changes of human serum albumin due to unsaturated fatty acid binding by chemical cross-linking and mass spectrometry. Biochem J 2005;387:695–702.

36. Fanali G, Fesce R, Agrati C, et al. Allosteric modulation of myristate and Mn(III) heme binding to human serum albumin. Optical and NMR spectroscopy characterization. FEBS J 2005;272:4672–83.

37. Brodersen R, Knudsen A, Pedersen AO. Cobinding of bilirubin and sulfonamide and of two bilirubin molecules to human serum albumin: a site model. Arch Biochem Biophys 1987;252:561–9.

38. Wennberg RP, Ahlfors CE, Rasmussen LF. The pathochemistry of kernicterus. Early Hum Dev 1979;3:353–72.

39. Klotz IM, Hunston DL. Protein affinities for small molecules: conceptions and misconceptions. Arch Biochem Biophys 1979;193:314–28.

40. Amin SB, Ahlfors CE. Bilirubin-binding capacity in premature infants. Pediatrics 2008;121:872–3 [author reply: 3].

41. Brodersen R, Funding L, Pedersen AO, et al. Binding of bilirubin to low-affinity sites of human serum albumin in vitro followed by co-crystallization. Scand J Clin Lab Invest 1972;29:433–46.

42. Amin SB, Lamola AA. Newborn jaundice technologies: unbound bilirubin and bilirubin binding capacity in neonates. Semin Perinatol 2011;35:134–40.

43. Koren R, Nissani E, Perlmutter-Hayman B. The kinetics of the reaction between bovine serum albumin and bilirubin. A second look. Biochim Biophys Acta 1982; 703:42–8.

44. Cashore WJ, Horwich A, Karotkin EH, et al. Influence of gestational age and clinical status on bilirubin-binding capacity in newborn infants. Sephadex G-25 gel filtration technique. Am J Dis Child 1977;131:898–901.

45. Cashore WJ. Free bilirubin concentrations and bilirubin-binding affinity in term and preterm infants. J Pediatr 1980;96:521–7.

46. Bender GJ, Cashore WJ, Oh W. Ontogeny of bilirubin-binding capacity and the effect of clinical status in premature infants born at less than 1300 grams. Pediatrics 2007;120:1067–73.

47. Lamola AA, Bhutani VK, Du L, et al. Neonatal bilirubin binding capacity discerns risk of neurological dysfunction. Pediatr Res 2015;77:334–9.

48. Cashore WJ, Horwich A, Laterra J, et al. Effect of postnatal age and clinical status of newborn infants on bilirubin-binding capacity. Biol Neonate 1977;32: 304–9.

49. Amin SB. Serial free bilirubin and bilirubin albumin binding affinity in premature infants. Proceedings of the Pediatric Academic Society Meeting; 2008:E-PAS 635844.11.

50. Cashore WJ, Oh W, Brodersen R. Reserve albumin and bilirubin toxicity index in infant serum. Acta Paediatr Scand 1983;72:415–9.

51. Meisel P, Jahrig D, Beyersdorff E, et al. Bilirubin binding and acid-base equilibrium in newborn infants with low birthweight. Acta Paediatr Scand 1988;77: 496–501.
52. Kozuki K, Oh W, Widness J, et al. Increase in bilirubin binding to albumin with correction of neonatal acidosis. Acta Paediatr Scand 1979;68:213–7.
53. Park W, Paust H, Schroder H. Lipid infusion in premature infants suffering from sepsis. JPEN J Parenter Enteral Nutr 1984;8:290–2.
54. Ebbesen F, Knudsen A. The risk of bilirubin encephalopathy, as estimated by plasma parameters, in neonates strongly suspected of having sepsis. Acta Paediatr 1993;82:26–9.
55. Ritter DA, Kenny JD, Norton HJ, et al. A prospective study of free bilirubin and other risk factors in the development of kernicterus in premature infants. Pediatrics 1982;69:260–6.
56. Kim MH, Yoon JJ, Sher J, et al. Lack of predictive indices in kernicterus: a comparison of clinical and pathologic factors in infants with or without kernicterus. Pediatrics 1980;66:852–8.
57. Turkel SB, Guttenberg ME, Moynes DR, et al. Lack of identifiable risk factors for kernicterus. Pediatrics 1980;66:502–6.
58. Itoh S, Yamakawa T, Onishi S, et al. The effect of bilirubin photoisomers on unbound-bilirubin concentrations estimated by the peroxidase method. Biochem J 1986;239:417–21.
59. Onishi S, Isobe K, Itoh S, et al. Metabolism of bilirubin and its photoisomers in newborn infants during phototherapy. J Biochem 1986;100:789–95.
60. McDonagh AF. Ex uno plures: the concealed complexity of bilirubin species in neonatal blood samples. Pediatrics 2006;118:1185–7.
61. Lamola AA, Flores J, Blumberg WE. Binding of photobilirubin to human serum albumin. Estimate of the affinity constant. Eur J Biochem 1983;132:165–9.
62. Meisel P, Biebler KE, Gens A, et al. Albumin binding of photobilirubin II. Biochem J 1983;213:25–9.
63. McDonagh AF, Vreman HJ, Wong RJ, et al. Photoisomers: obfuscating factors in clinical peroxidase measurements of unbound bilirubin? Pediatrics 2009;123: 67–76.
64. Itoh S, Kawada K, Kusaka T, et al. Influence of glucuronosyl bilirubin and (EZ)-cyclobilirubin on determination of serum unbound bilirubin by UB-analyser. Ann Clin Biochem 2002;39:583–8.
65. Ebbesen F, Jacobsen J. Bilirubin-albumin binding affinity and serum albumin concentration during intensive phototherapy (blue double light) in jaundiced newborn infants. Eur J Pediatr 1980;134:261–3.
66. Nakamura H, Lee Y, Uetani Y, et al. Effects of phototherapy on serum unbound bilirubin i icteric newborn infants. Biol Neonate 1981;39:295–9.
67. Myara A, Sender A, Valette V, et al. Early changes in cutaneous bilirubin and serum bilirubin isomers during intensive phototherapy of jaundiced neonates with blue and green light. Biol Neonate 1997;71:75–82.
68. Brodersen R. Competitive binding of bilirubin and drugs to human serum albumin studied by enzymatic oxidation. J Clin Invest 1974;54:1353–64.
69. Robertson A, Karp W, Brodersen R. Bilirubin displacing effect of drugs used in neonatology. Acta Paediatr Scand 1991;80:1119–27.
70. Wadsworth SJ, Suh B. In vitro displacement of bilirubin by antibiotics and 2-hydroxybenzoylglycine in newborns. Antimicrob Agents Chemother 1988; 32:1571–5.

71. Funato M, Lee Y, Onishi S, et al. Influence of drugs on albumin and bilirubin interaction. Acta Paediatr Jpn 1989;31:35–44.

72. Maruyama K, Harada S, Nishigori H, et al. Classification of drugs on the basis of bilirubin-displacing effect on human serum albumin. Chem Pharm Bull 1984;32: 2414–20.

73. Ambat MT, Ostrea EM Jr, Aranda JV. Effect of ibuprofen L-lysinate on bilirubin binding to albumin as measured by saturation index and horseradish peroxidase assays. J Perinatol 2008;28:287–90.

74. Ahlfors CE. Effect of ibuprofen on bilirubin-albumin binding. J Pediatr 2004;144: 386–8.

75. Cooper-Peel C, Brodersen R, Robertson A. Does ibuprofen affect bilirubin-albumin binding in newborn infant serum? Pharmacol Toxicol 1996;79:297–9.

76. Amin SB, Miravalle N. Effect of ibuprofen on bilirubin-albumin binding affinity in premature infants. J Perinat Med 2011;39:55–8.

77. Desfrere L, Thibaut C, Kibleur Y, et al. Unbound bilirubin does not increase during ibuprofen treatment of patent ductus arteriosus in preterm infants. J Pediatr 2012;160:258–64.e1.

78. Aranda JV, Varvarigou A, Beharry K, et al. Pharmacokinetics and protein binding of intravenous ibuprofen in the premature newborn infant. Acta Paediatr 1997; 86:289–93.

79. Andrew G, Chan G, Schiff D. Lipid metabolism in the neonate. II. The effect of Intralipid on bilirubin binding in vitro and in vivo. J Pediatr 1976;88:279–84.

80. Shennan AT, Bryan MH, Angel A. The effect of gestational age on intralipid tolerance in newborn infants. J Pediatr 1977;91:134–7.

81. Ruben S, Kleinfeld AM, Richeiri GV, et al. Serum levels of unbound free fatty acids. II: the effect of intralipid administration in premature infants. J Am Coll Nutr 1997;16:85–7.

82. Ostrea EM Jr, Bassel M, Fleury CA, et al. Influence of free fatty acids and glucose infusion on serum bilirubin and bilirubin binding to albumin: clinical implications. J Pediatr 1983;102:426–32.

83. Odell GB, Cukier JO, Ostrea EM Jr, et al. The influence of fatty acids on the binding of bilirubin to albumin. J Lab Clin Med 1977;89:295–307.

84. Berde CB, Hudson BS, Simoni RD, et al. Human serum albumin. Spectroscopic studies of binding and proximity relationships for fatty acids and bilirubin. J Biol Chem 1979;254:391–400.

85. Thiessen H, Jacobsen J, Brodersen R. Displacement of albumin-bound bilirubin by fatty acids. Acta Paediatr Scand 1972;61:285–8.

86. Whitington PF, Burckart GJ, Gross SR, et al. Alterations in reserve bilirubin binding capacity of albumin by free fatty acids. II. In vitro and in vivo studies using difference spectroscopy. J Pediatr Gastroenterol Nutr 1982;1:495–501.

87. Starinsky R, Shafrir E. Displacement of albumin-bound bilirubin by free fatty acids. Implications for neonatal hyperbilirubinemia. Clin Chim Acta 1970;29: 311–8.

88. Chan G, Schiff D, Stern L. Competitive binding of free fatty acids and bilirubin to albumin: differences in HBABA dye versus sephadex G-25 interpretation of results. Clin Biochem 1971;4:208–14.

89. Brans YW, Ritter DA, Kenny JD, et al. Influence of intravenous fat emulsion on serum bilirubin in very low birthweight neonates. Arch Dis Child 1987;62: 156–60.

90. Spear ML, Stahl GE, Paul MH, et al. The effect of 15-hour fat infusions of varying dosage on bilirubin binding to albumin. JPEN J Parenter Enteral Nutr 1985;9: 144–7.

91. Rubin M, Harell D, Naor N, et al. Lipid infusion with different triglyceride cores (long-chain vs medium-chain/long-chain triglycerides): effect on plasma lipids and bilirubin binding in premature infants. JPEN J Parenter Enteral Nutr 1991;15:642–6.

92. Amin SB, Harte T, Scholer L, et al. Intravenous lipid and bilirubin-albumin binding variables in premature infants. Pediatrics 2009;124:211–7.

93. Amin SB. Effect of free fatty acids on bilirubin-albumin binding affinity and unbound bilirubin in premature infants. JPEN J Parenter Enteral Nutr 2010;34:414–20.

94. Cashore WJ, Oh W. Unbound bilirubin and kernicterus in low-birth-weight infants. Pediatrics 1982;69:481–5.

95. Amin SB, Ahlfors C, Orlando MS, et al. Bilirubin and serial auditory brainstem responses in premature infants. Pediatrics 2001;107:664–70.

96. Iskander I, Gamaleldin R, El Houchi S, et al. Serum bilirubin and bilirubin/albumin ratio as predictors of bilirubin encephalopathy. Pediatrics 2014;134:e1330–9.

97. Hulzebos CV, Dijk PH, van Imhoff DE, et al. The bilirubin albumin ratio in the management of hyperbilirubinemia in preterm infants to improve neurodevelopmental outcome: a randomized controlled trial – BARTrial. PLoS One 2014;9:e99466.

98. Govaert P, Lequin M, Swarte R, et al. Changes in globus pallidus with (pre)term kernicterus. Pediatrics 2003;112:1256–63.

99. Valaes T, Kapitulnik J, Kaufmann NA, et al. Experience with Sephadex gel filtration in assessing the risk of bilirubin encephalopathy in neonatal jaundice. Birth Defects Orig Artic Ser 1976;12:215–28.

100. Kapitulnik J, Valaes T, Kaufmann NA, et al. Clinical evaluation of Sephadex gel filtration in estimation of bilirubin binding in serum in neonatal jaundice. Arch Dis Child 1974;49:886–94.

101. Zamet P, Nakamura H, Perez-Robles S, et al. The use of critical levels of birth weight and "free bilirubin" as an approach for prevention of kernicterus. Biol Neonate 1975;26:274–82.

102. Odell GB, Storey GN, Rosenberg LA. Studies in kernicterus. 3. The saturation of serum proteins with bilirubin during neonatal life and its relationship to brain damage at five years. J Pediatr 1970;76:12–21.

103. Waters WJ, Porter E. Indications for exchange transfusion based upon the role of albumin in the treatment of hemolytic disease of the newborn. Pediatrics 1964;33:749–57.

104. Jacobsen J, Wennberg RP. Determination of unbound bilirubin in the serum of newborns. Clin Chem 1974;20:783.

105. Nakamura H, Yonetani M, Uetani Y, et al. Determination of serum unbound bilirubin for prediction of kernicterus in low birthweight infants. Acta Paediatr Jap 1992;34:642–7.

106. Ahlfors CE, Amin SB, Parker AE. Unbound bilirubin predicts abnormal automated auditory brainstem response in a diverse newborn population. J Perinatol 2009; 29:305–9.

107. Amin SB, Wang H, Laroia N, et al. Unbound bilirubin and auditory neuropathy spectrum disorder in late preterm and term infants with severe jaundice. The Journal of Pediatrics 2016, in press.

108. Oh W, Stevenson DK, Tyson JE, et al. Influence of clinical status on the association between plasma total and unbound bilirubin and death or adverse neurodevelopmental outcomes in extremely low birth weight infants. Acta Paediatr 2010;99:673–8.

A Pharmacologic View of Phototherapy

Angelo A. Lamola, PhD*

KEYWORDS

- Phototherapy • Molecular mechanisms of phototherapy
- Pharmacology of phototherapy

KEY POINTS

- By considering the photons of therapy light as molecules of a drug, this view connects therapeutic efficacy with photon wavelength, photon dose, dose rate and regimen, efficiency of photon absorption by bilirubin, quantum yields of photoproducts, and their metabolic courses.
- Based on this view, recommendations to ultimately improve efficacy and safety are presented.
- Special attention is given to phototherapy regimens for low gestational age, low birthweight infants.

INTRODUCTION

Because of its efficacy in reducing the need for exchange transfusion, the concomitant reduction in the incidence of kernicterus, and its apparent safety, noninvasive phototherapy to reduce the body burden of unconjugated bilirubin has been widely used for nearly 5 decades.[1–6] However, it is now opined that phototherapy may be overprescribed.[7]

The initial 1957 phototherapy unit[8,9] used an adapted blue light source mostly conforming to the absorption spectrum of bilirubin and avoidance of harmful ultraviolet (UV) light. The use of blue light by these pioneers was consistent with the directive of the first symposium held in 1969,[10] which was intended to devise recommendations for the clinical application of phototherapy, to involve judgments similar to those made in deciding on the clinical use of a new drug. However, aside from general recommendations that have withstood the test of time,[2,3,10] there are no specific standards for phototherapy practice, and a pharmacologic approach to its use remains

Disclosure: The author has no financial relationships and conflicts of interest to this article. This article was supported in part by the Ahlfors Center for Unbound Bilirubin Research & Development and the Kaplan-Goldstein Family Foundation.
Division of Neonatal and Developmental Medicine, Department of Pediatrics, Stanford University School of Medicine, Stanford, CA, USA
* 750 Welch Road, Suite #315, Palo Alto, CA 94304.
E-mail address: aalsml@msn.com

incomplete. The reasons for this practice gap include (1) the inability to adequately compare studies using different light sources and regimens, (2) the vagaries of spectroradiometrics, (3) the complexities of chemistry of the photoproducts of bilirubin and their therapeutic roles, (4) insufficient attention given to the optical properties of neonatal skin, and (5) the limited knowledge of the dynamics of the phototherapy processes. Without attention to efficiency or possible harm, the use of any light source (fluorescent, halogen, light-emitting diodes [LEDs], or even the sun) of sufficient intensity in the 450-nm to 500-nm range over a sufficient skin area can reduce the total serum/plasma bilirubin (TB) level in an infant, often at a clinically useful rate. There are a myriad of phototherapy devices and regimens in clinical use that are evidently providing more good than harm. However, in the spirit of primum non nocere, there is an obligation to improve the risk/benefit ratio of phototherapy to deliver the most effective and safest care.

Phototherapy is a multistep biomolecular process. It works by creating pathways for excretion of bilirubin without conjugation of the toxic pigment. The general outline of the processes of phototherapy established by 1985[11] remains valid. Absorption of light by bilirubin in vivo leads primarily to 2 types of molecular alterations: configurational (Z to E or cis to trans) and structural (vide infra) isomerizations. These photoproducts differ in their (1) rates of production depending on exposure light; (2) modes and rates of excretion; and (3) stabilities. Integration of this knowledge into a dynamic model to optimize risk/benefit presents a difficult exercise in process simulation that should, however, be attempted. Short of a totally integrated model, several clinically relevant conclusions can be drawn from partial integrations. For example, factors that control therapeutically useful absorption of exposure light by bilirubin, the sine qua non of phototherapy, are now well described[12] and should be embodied in a standard regimen.

This article provides physics-based, chemistry-based, and physiology-based descriptions of the phototherapy processes as a basis to interpret clinical observations. Suggestions for improved regimens are made when possible, and knowledge gaps for optimizing risk/benefit ratios based on pharmacologic rigor are identified. As much as is allowed by current knowledge, reference is made to the special needs of premature infants.

Currently recommended prescriptions and regimens for phototherapy are well reviewed in recent reports[13–15] and are not repeated here. Also not reviewed is the literature relating phototherapy to reduced bilirubin toxicity[16] and suspected phototherapy side effects.[17]

Light, Photons, Light Absorption, and Photochemistry: Photons as Drug Units

Light is that form of energy transported as an electromagnetic wave. The wavelength range of visible light is about 400 to 700 nm. Humans' perception of light as a continuous energy stream belies that it is composed of discrete packets of energy called photons. The energy (E) carried by a photon is inversely proportional to the wavelength. Accordingly, a 400-nm photon (blue) contains about 25% more energy than one at 500 nm (visibly green). That is, for the same light dose measured in energy units (eg, μW-h), there are 20% more photons at 500 nm than at 400 nm. Therefore, to compare the effectiveness of light of different wavelengths to cause some effect, it is necessary to consider the difference in measuring the light by dose energy or by photon count.

The sine qua non of photochemistry is the absorption of light and its associated energy. In phototherapy, the effective light is directly absorbed by bilirubin. The absorption spectrum is a plot of the probability of absorption versus the wavelength. **Fig. 1** shows the absorption spectra of bilirubin (Z,Z-IXα) and hemoglobin (Hb).

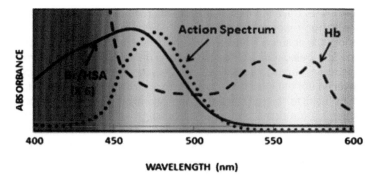

Fig. 1. Absorption spectra of hemoglobin (Hb) and bilirubin in human serum albumin (Br/HSA). The relative absorption strength of Hb and bilirubin for blood with TB = 10 mg/dL and Hct = 50%. The bilirubin absorption is magnified by a factor of 6 for easier visualization. The "action spectrum" is the relative fraction of the light absorbed by bilirubin, $\approx$5% at the maximum (476 nm), for TB = 10 mg/dL and hematocrit (Hct) = 50%.

Bilirubin absorbs light in the blue portion of the visible spectrum (as well as in the non-visible UV region). Thus, in white light, bilirubin appears yellow-orange. Hb absorbs light with even higher probability where bilirubin absorbs. The spectra of complex molecules are smeared out and appear as broad bands because of the vibrations, the various possible geometries, and the environments of the molecules, which modulate the wavelengths that can be absorbed. The spectrum shown in **Fig. 1** is that of bilirubin bound to human serum albumin, which is the form of virtually all of the bilirubin in blood. The spectrum of bilirubin in other environments can be significantly different.

Consider the analogy of photons to molecules of a drug. Analogous to designing the molecular structure of a drug to interact with a specific biomolecular entity, the wavelength of light can be chosen for absorption by specific target molecules. Additional specificity of the wavelength range may be dictated by needs, such as the avoidance of untoward side effects. For example, bilirubin absorbs UV light, as do almost all biomolecules such as proteins and nucleic acids. UV light absorption by the latter can lead to deleterious effects. Because nucleic acids and proteins without prosthetic groups (eg, heme) do not absorb blue light, it is possible to have blue light absorbed by bilirubin without affecting proteins and nucleic acids. No phototherapy devices marketed in the United States expose infants to UV light.

The total number of therapeutic photons to which a molecular target is exposed is analogous to the dose of a drug. The intensity or irradiance (photons per unit time) of the light is analogous to the drug dose rate. Although light dose and irradiance are most conveniently measured in units of energy and energy per unit time, respectively, understanding light-driven molecular processes requires the counting of photons because photochemistry is initiated by absorption of single photons by single molecules.

The average 8-hour dose (108 mg) of 7 common antibiotics (eg, ampicillin) used in the neonatal intensive care unit[18] provides 1.4×10^{20} molecules of the drug based on an average molecular weight of 460 g/mole. In comparison, at a common irradiance (30 μW/cm^2/nm) of phototherapy over 1000 cm^2 of skin surface for 8 hours, an LED light source with peak wavelength at 475 nm provides 2×10^{23} photons. The number of bilirubin molecules in circulation and in the extravascular compartment of a 3-kg infant with a hematocrit (Hct) of 50%, and a TB of 15 mg/dL is roughly 4×10^{19} molecules (40 mg). Thus, there would be 5000 photons available per circulating bilirubin molecule to drive the therapeutic effect. That this is consistent with the efficacy of phototherapy is elucidated later.

When a molecule absorbs a photon, the photon's energy is transferred to its electrons. The resultant electronically excited state is unstable. Competing processes by which the molecule returns to a stable state include reemission of the energy (luminescence), conversion of the electronic energy into vibrational energy (heat) followed by transfer of the heat to its surroundings, and chemical alteration (photochemistry). The photochemical products are usually produced with excess vibrational energy (heat) that is also transferred to the surroundings. Unless the excited molecule reemits a photon with high efficiency, the energy of the absorbed photon is mostly converted to heat. The analogy between therapeutic photons and molecular drugs therefore fails in an important regard: absorption of light leads to heat deposition.[12] At present, the risk/benefit ratio of such heat transfer to a newborn, especially a small low gestational age (GA) and/or sick newborn, is not well understood.

Management of Unconjugated Neonatal Hyperbilirubinemia: Indications for Phototherapy

The goal of the management of neonatal unconjugated hyperbilirubinemia is to keep the infant's body burden of bilirubin at a level at which the risk for developing bilirubin neurotoxicity is low. However, in the assessment of risk, fundamental gaps remain regarding the mechanism of neurotoxicity,[19] the measure of the body burden of bilirubin, and the definition of a safe level of bilirubin.[1,20] Direct neurologic measures of bilirubin toxicity have remained elusive.[19] To make prescription of therapies precise warrants an individualized evidence-based risk assessment paradigm[20–22] to replace the current consensus-based TB thresholds for phototherapy and exchange transfusion–based GA, clinical signs of hemolysis, and the bilirubin/albumin molar ratio (BAMR).[2,3,23,24] As discussed later, an optimized individualized regimen for phototherapy should also take into account an infant's starting TB, a quantitative estimate of bilirubin production rate, the safe TB goal, and the speed at which the safe TB needs to be attained.

Body burden of bilirubin

The default measure of the burden of unconjugated bilirubin on which clinical practice is based is the TB concentration (minus the direct bilirubin). TB may not reflect the body burden of bilirubin for several reasons. TB does not reflect differences in the amount of bilirubin in the serum pool for the range of Hct's in newborns per se. Consider 2 infants of similar weight and blood volumes: an infant with an Hct of 40% would have 1.5 times the amount (weight) of serum bilirubin as an infant with an Hct of 60% for the same TB level. Note that levels of toxins are generally expressed as weight of toxin per kilogram of body weight (BW).

Other bilirubin pools include extravascular albumin-bound bilirubin, and bilirubin in red blood cells and tissue, which can both become significant when the bilirubin-albumin binding capacity (BBC) is approached. Given sufficiently rapid equilibration of these pools with the serum bilirubin, they could be proportionate to the TB. However, the accumulation of bilirubin in tissue when BBC is approached and the possible increase in risk for neurotoxicity with the time an infant's TB remains near the BBC have not been elucidated. As phototherapy-mediated excretion or exchange transfusion reduces TB, this extravascular bilirubin can reenter circulation.

Bilirubin/albumin binding status

Almost all of the bilirubin in serum is strongly, but reversibly, bound to its transport protein, albumin. The BBC of albumin controls a dynamic relationship between the levels of bound and unbound (free) bilirubin (UB) and the ability to tolerate increasing bilirubin loads.[20,23] However, BBC is not consonant with the albumin level. The ability of albumin to bind bilirubin is confounded by molecular, biological, and metabolic factors, including an infant's GA and the presence of competitive antagonists. UB crosses membranes effectively and enters cells. The cellular uptake of bilirubin seems to be a reversible passive process such that bilirubin can be extracted from cells by increased extracellular BBC.[2,20,23]

Clinical assays of TB, UB, albumin, BBC, and calculated BAMR together with BW, GA, postnatal age, and observations of concurrent hemolysis, sepsis, and rate of TB increase have been considered in neurotoxicity risk assessment.[2,3] However, their individual and combined predictive utility has yet to be refined. However, it seems that increased risk at a lower GA is primarily caused by an associated lower BBC.[23] Availability of facile point-of-care assays of BBC (and UB) may provide the confidence to forego phototherapy for hyperbilirubinemic term and near-term infants with high BBC levels, or consideration to initiate phototherapy earlier for infants with modest TB but low BBC.[23,24]

Measures of phototherapy efficacy

Clinical efficacy of phototherapy refers to the timely reduction of TB to a safe level for an individual infant. Current guidelines[2,3,13] are meant to ensure such and suggest that, in general, an effective phototherapy regimen should reduce TB by 3 or 4 mg/dL within 8 to 12 hours. Most studies of phototherapy optimization measured the TB reduction after fixed durations of phototherapy, commonly after 24 hours. Because the rate of decrease can change significantly (vide infra) over time, the 24-hour point may not relate to the factor intended for optimization. In any case, the change in TB may not adequately reflect the change in the body burden of bilirubin.

Significant for comparisons of studies of phototherapy, especially at different sites, is uncertainty in assessing differences in light sources (wavelength ranges) and radiometry (no standard methodology) caused by inadequate descriptions. Proper comparisons also require translations between irradiance measured in energy units and photon count.[12] The recent use of LED sources with easily adjusted irradiance, and more standardized radiometry, make it easier to integrate and/or compare data from different studies. However, there is not yet sufficient attention to other phototherapy parameters now known to require consideration. These parameters include an infant's Hb level, starting TB, BW, and GA (related to bilirubin production rate), and the presence of hemolysis.

Optical Properties of Neonatal Skin: Action Spectrum and Hematocrit Dependence of Phototherapy

Skin optics

Knowledge of salient optical properties of the neonatal skin is necessary to interpret clinical observations of phototherapy. Recently, knowledge of the optical properties of neonatal skin[25,26] obtained for development of transcutaneous bilirubinometry has been applied to phototherapy.[12] The simple model obtained is shown in **Fig. 2**.

Light in the range of 400 to 520 nm entering the epidermis is mostly transmitted. Some back-scatter occurs as well as absorption by melanin. Both back-scatter and melanin absorbance have weak wavelength dependences in the range, so the epidermis can be considered a neutral density filter. Back-scatter from the epidermis and dermis amounts to less than 7% of the impinging light. At a melanosome content of 10% volume/volume, a high value for even a neonate with increased melanin pigmentation, absorbance by melanin only reduces phototherapy efficacy by less

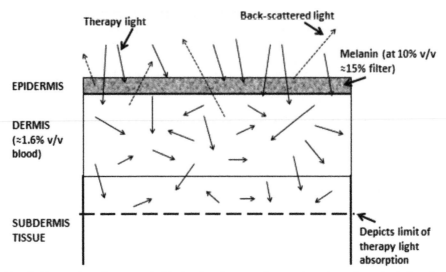

Fig. 2. The optics of neonatal skin in the therapeutic wavelength region, depicting the immediate diffusion of the light in the dermis and the total absorbance of exposure light within the dermis and nearby subdermis caused by the high absorbance by Hb there.

than 15%. The size distribution and varied refractive indices of structural elements of the dermis and subdermal tissue cause rampant diffusive light scattering in skin even for low GA neonates. Because of the rich vasculature of the dermis, Hb is by far the major absorber of visible light in that part of the skin. Other pigments that can have significant absorbance at increased levels include bilirubin and carotenoids. Light absorption by other endogenous pigments is usually insignificant.

Together, the vascular structure and light diffusion in the dermis provide a key simplification: light absorption and the distributions of Hb and bilirubin can be considered homogeneous, which allows the facile calculation of the fraction of exposure light at any wavelength that is absorbed by bilirubin under the assumptions that no other significant absorbing species are present except Hb and bilirubin, and that greater than 90% of the light entering the dermis is absorbed there and in the nearby subdermis. The latter assumption is justified by the strong absorbance of Hb and the high blood content of neonatal skin ($\approx$2% volume/volume).[27] Neonates at lower GAs have thinner dermis, but a compensating higher blood content and flow.

Action spectrum

Using this model, the fractions of exposure light absorbed by bilirubin for ranges of TB (5–25 mg/dL), Hct (20%–70%), and Hb oxygenation (60%–90%), with back-scatter and melanin were calculated.[12] The wavelength for maximum bilirubin absorbance for all the cases varies only between 475 and 478 nm. This small variance is caused by the dominance of competition of Hb with bilirubin for the light. Because phototherapy is driven by light absorbed by bilirubin, a spectrum of the fraction of exposure light absorbed by bilirubin calculated in this way (see **Fig. 1**; **Fig. 3**) should represent a first-order action spectrum for phototherapy. (An action spectrum represents the extent or effectiveness of a light-driven process as a function of the wavelength.) This action spectrum, which is essentially in the range 460 to 490 nm, is substantially different from the absorption spectrum of bilirubin bound to albumin. Light of wavelengths outside this range is predominantly absorbed by Hb and uselessly heats the infant.[12]

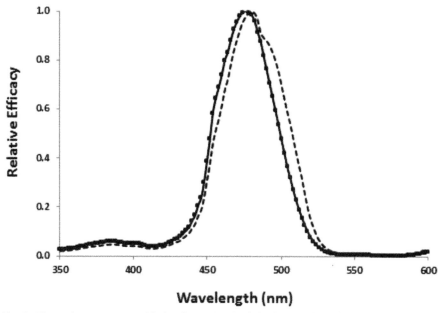

Fig. 3. The action spectrum of light absorption by bilirubin in blood for a range of TB and Hct's expected in hyperbilirubinemic newborns (*solid line*). This spectrum is not altered by inclusion of back-scattering or melanin absorption by the skin (*dotted line*). If the production of lumirubin were responsible for all of the phototherapy effect the spectrum would be slightly shifted toward higher wavelengths (*dashed line*).

Also shown in **Fig. 3** is the calculated action spectrum for the extreme case in which the structural isomer photoproduct (lumirubin; vide infra) is the sole contributor to the phototherapy effect. This spectrum is shifted to higher wavelengths by only about 3 nm and is slightly broadened.

Many clinical studies to discern the most effective light sources for phototherapy have been reported over the years.[28,29] It is difficult to compare the data in a quantitative manner because of different regimens used, lack of light source spectra and radiometric detail, the diverse assessments of phototherapy efficacy, and the lack of control of parameters such as starting TB, Hb, and Hct. However, the overall impression is that blue-green light that is therapy light peaked at a longer wavelength than the bilirubin-albumin absorption maximum, is most effective. More recent clinical studies with better controls have reinforced this conclusion.[30] Findings are consistent with the action spectrum described earlier. Increased effectiveness of blue-green compared with blue light is not, per se, because of the often-stated deeper penetration of blue-green light, but because bilirubin competes best with Hb for light absorption in that spectral region.

Hematocrit dependence
A corollary of the predominance of light absorption by Hb in the therapeutic range is a predicted dependence of phototherapy efficacy on the Hb level or the Hct: the higher the Hct, the lower the expected efficacy.[12] For an equal starting level of TB, and all else being equal, the rate of bilirubin photoalteration in an infant with an Hct of 60% is calculated to be 33% lower than that for an infant with an Hct of 40%. This

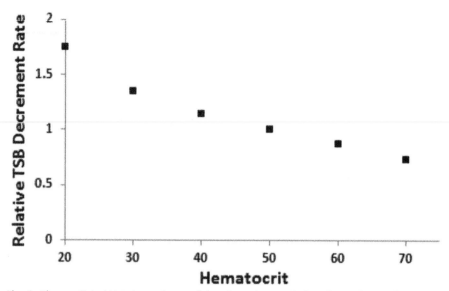

Fig. 4. The predicted Hct dependence of the phototherapy-induced initial rate of TB reduction for equal irradiance and starting TB. The arbitrary value (1.0) at Hct = 50% is chosen for easy comparison. The Hct dependence is close to linear over the clinically relevant range (30% to 70%). TSB, total serum bilirubin.

dependence is shown in **Fig. 4**. The Hct dependence of bilirubin photoalteration has been shown in vitro[31] and the effect is also observed in vivo.[32]

Bilirubin: Structure, Properties, and Photochemistry

Because of the complex structure and bothersome physical and chemical properties of bilirubin, the elucidation of its photochemistry has been painstaking. The history of this endeavor has recently been thoroughly documented by Dr. David A. Lightner.[33] Only those features particularly germane to phototherapy are described in an extremely abridged manner here.

4Z,15Z-bilirubin

A structure of 4Z,15Z (unconjugated) bilirubin produced from normal heme catabolism is shown in **Fig. 5A** in the iconic conformation that rationalizes so much of what is known about neonatal hyperbilirubinemia and phototherapy. The 2 double bonds at positions 4 and 15 can have the groups attached to them either in the Z (zusammen, meaning same side) or E (entgegen, meaning opposite side) configurations. In the Z,Z configuration, bilirubin can fold into a conformation in which all of the polar groups of the molecule are internally hydrogen bonded and sequestered from its solvent environment. This conformation explains the extremely low water solubility of bilirubin and its lipophilic nature, which allows it to reside in and cross lipid membranes. It explains why it requires transport and its specific binding by albumin, and why it requires conjugation with water-solubilizing groups to effect excretion.

Configurational isomers (E isomers)

When bilirubin absorbs a photon its electronic structure is altered, weakening the double bonds at positions 4 and 15, and allowing a twisting around one or the other of these bonds. This twisting can occur quickly, within picoseconds for

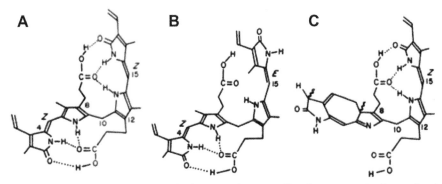

Fig. 5. Structures of: (A) *4Z,15Z*-bilirubin-IXα, showing all polar groups in the molecule having internal hydrogen bonds; (B) *4Z,15E*-bilirubin, showing that the E configuration precludes half of the internal hydrogen bonding; and (C) lumirubin, showing that internal hydrogen bonding of all polar groups is precluded in this structural isomer.

bilirubin in chloroform.[34] The excited molecule relaxes, reforming the double bond with either return to the Z configuration or isomerization to the E configuration. Both *4Z,15E*-bilirubin and *4E,15Z*-bilirubin are formed in chloroform solution. Isomerization is more restricted for bilirubin bound to albumin. The binding is specific such that the 4 end is held more tightly than the 15 end and results in nearly exclusive formation of *4Z,15E*-bilirubin (**Fig. 5B**). The probability that the twisted excited bilirubin on albumin relaxes to *4Z,15E*-bilirubin is about 20%,[34] which means that the initial quantum yield (isomers formed per photon absorbed) is about 0.2, which is very high. When the E isomer absorbs light, the same twisting can occur, and the isomerization can be reversed. With continued irradiation of bilirubin-albumin an equilibrium mixture, the photostationary state (pss), of bilirubin and *4Z,15E*-bilirubin is reached. The E configurations and bilirubin have similar, but not identical, absorption spectra and so the pss ratio varies from 20% to 30% for different exposure wavelengths.

Albumin binding slows the twisting rate of the excited bilirubin to allow a small fraction (0.1%) to reemit a photon as fluorescence. It is this fluorescence that is used as the basis for hematofluorometric assays of TB and BBC.[35] In a frozen matrix, where twisting is precluded, the fluorescence yield is nearly 100%.[34]

Because of its high quantum yield, *4Z,15E*-bilirubin is rapidly accumulated and, at commonly used irradiances, the pss can be reached in the blood of infants within a few hours of phototherapy.[36] Once the pss is reached, absorbed light just shuttles the configurations back and forth and is wasted with regard to phototherapy. To maintain the pss, it is sufficient at that point to reduce the irradiance to that sufficient to isomerize any newly produced bilirubin. Photoreversibility of configurational isomerization has implications for cycled phototherapy (vide infra).

4Z,15E-bilirubin cannot form a completely internally hydrogen-bonded structure as does bilirubin, and so it is more polar and water soluble than bilirubin. This property allows direct excretion of *4Z,15E*-bilirubin into the bile without conjugation in the liver.[37] The excretion is fast in Gunn rats but very slow in humans.[37,38] *4Z,15E*-bilirubin is not distinguished from bilirubin by the common diazo and colorimetric assays.

E isomers can revert to more thermodynamically stable Z isomers by thermal (not involving light) routes that can be acid/base catalyzed. *4Z,15E*-bilirubin binds strongly to albumin, stabilizing it toward thermal reversion. Little *4Z,15E*-bilirubin compared with bilirubin is found in the bile of infants under phototherapy and it is conjectured that, after excretion into bile, it reverts to bilirubin.[36,39]

Lumirubin

Photoexcited bilirubin undergoes another kind of isomerization in which the double-bonded carbon atoms on one end ring form new bonds with atoms in the adjacent ring-forming isomers, collectively called lumirubin (**Fig. 5**C).[39,40] The quantum yield of formation of lumirubin from bilirubin bound to albumin is about 0.0015, or more than 100 times lower than the yield of 4Z,15E-bilirubin.[41] There is no delay in the production of lumirubin, which indicates that it is formed directly from bilirubin and not from 4Z,15E-bilirubin (DT Linfield, 2015, unpublished data). The quantum yield has a substantial wavelength dependence increasing by nearly a factor of 3, going from 450 to 500 nm.[41] Lumirubin does not revert to bilirubin with light and is also thermally stable.[11,39,40] Like the other isomers, lumirubin binds to albumin.

Although lumirubin is formed much more slowly than 4Z,15E-bilirubin, the latter does not increase past the pss, and so, with continued irradiation, lumirubin accumulates and, in vitro, can become the dominant photoproduct.[39,40] Lumirubin is not detected by the common diazo assays. It can be assayed by liquid chromatography in the serum/plasma of infants under phototherapy and reaches levels of more than 4% of the TB. Lumirubin is more polar and as water soluble as 4Z,15E-bilirubin and is excreted into the bile without hepatic conjugation at a much faster rate than is 4Z,15E-bilirubin.[42] Lumirubin is stable in the bile and does not seem to reenter the circulation.[39,40]

Photo-oxidation products

In the presence of oxygen, photodegradation of bilirubin to low molecular weight, colorless products is observed in vitro, and similar products have been observed in vivo.[43,44] However, the rate of this oxidative degradation in vivo is very low, by a factor of one-hundredth to one-thousandth, compared with the isomerizations. These degradation products are easily excreted in urine.[44] However, this low-efficiency chemistry is not significant for the therapeutic effect of phototherapy. The formation of these products in vivo indicates possible oxidative stress associated with phototherapy (vide infra).

Excretion Rates of Photoproducts: Relative Roles in Phototherapy

Unless otherwise indicated, estimations presented later in this article assume an Hct of 50%, and the use of narrow-bandwidth LEDs centered at 475 nm, a model LED source (mLED). In the remainder of this article, Z,E-bilirubin is used as shorthand for 4Z,15E-bilirubin.

Z,E-bilirubin excretion

The average half-life of Z,E-bilirubin determined in serial serum samples from infants after phototherapy cessation is about 13 hours (recalculated from original data).[38] The rate constant is therefore about 0.06 per hour. It is assumed that this disappearance of Z,E-bilirubin is caused by direct excretion.

Z,E-bilirubin is the predominant configurational isomer in vivo; other E isomers are ignored in the following estimations. Depending on the light source and irradiance, the photostationary (pss) fraction of 20% to 30% Z,E-bilirubin can be achieved in about 1 hour of phototherapy. For the mLED source, the pss has 25% Z,E-bilirubin. Ignoring the small amounts of other photoproducts, the Z,E-bilirubin represents 25% of the TB, and so the rate of excretion is 0.06 × 25% or 1.5% per hour of the TB. Continued phototherapy at sufficient irradiance will maintain the Z,E-bilirubin level at about 25% of the TB and an excretion rate of about 1.5% per hour of the TB. At a TB of 20 mg/dL, the rate is 0.3 mg/dL/h; at a TB of 5 mg/dL, it is only 0.08 mg/dL/h.

Because *Z,E*-bilirubin reverts to bilirubin in the bile, a portion may be reabsorbed into circulation, reducing the net rate of excretion. The 1.5% per hour of TB should be taken as an upper limit for the rate of phototherapy-mediated excretion via the *Z,E*-bilirubin mechanism.

Lumirubin excretion

The average half-life of lumirubin in sera of neonates after cessation of phototherapy is observed to be 1.9 hours,[42] corresponding with a rate constant of 0.38 per hour. The lumirubin excretion rate is the lumirubin level times the rate constant, 0.38 per hour. Because lumirubin formation is not photoreversible, the amount of lumirubin in the serum depends on the irradiance in competition with lumirubin excretion; therefore, the higher the irradiance, the greater the level of lumirubin.

In the same study,[42] the average lumirubin level after continuous phototherapy for a few hours was found to be 3.2% of the TB. Assuming that this represents balance of production and excretion rates, the excretion rate is calculated to be 1.2% per hour of the TB. From these data, the rates of photoproduction and excretion can be estimated for other light sources, irradiances, and TB levels to estimate the relative importance of the *Z,E*-bilirubin and lumirubin routes.

Configurational versus structural isomerization

Although recent reviews of phototherapy leave open the question of whether the *Z,E*-bilirubin or lumirubin route is the more important, the emphasis placed on the faster excretion rate of lumirubin and possible frustration of the *Z,E*-bilirubin route caused by reabsorption imply a strong bias toward the lumirubin route.[5,13,14] As postulated later, depending on the irradiance and TB level, the rates of the 2 routes for phototherapy-mediated excretion can be comparable.

The data described earlier were used to estimate phototherapy-mediated excretion rates expressed as the per-hour exit of bilirubin isomers observed in the serum/plasma. The TB levels chosen reflect action levels that could pertain for lower-GA neonates. The rates given in **Table 1** may not be quantitatively correct. However, the relative values are instructive. Assuming the pss is reached quickly, the *Z,E*-bilirubin excretion rate

Table 1
Relative initial rates of phototherapy-mediated excretion pathways expressed as the excretion of bilirubin isomers into bile per hour

Irradiance (μW/cm^2/nm)	TB (mg/dL)	Excretion Rate (mg/dL/h) Via:		
		Z,E-bilirubin	Lumirubin	*Z,E*-bilirubin + Lumirubin
10	5	0.08	0.06	0.14
	8	0.13	0.10	0.23
	10	0.16	0.12	0.28
	15	0.24	0.18	0.42
20	5	0.08	0.12	0.20
	8	0.13	0.20	0.33
	10	0.16	0.24	0.40
	15	0.24	0.36	0.60
30	5	0.08	0.18	0.26
	8	0.13	0.30	0.43
	10	0.16	0.36	0.52
	15	0.24	0.54	0.78

These rates are not net decrements because they do not reflect any bilirubin reentering the blood from extravascular compartments or new bilirubin formation from heme catabolism.

is independent of the irradiance for constant TB. In contrast, the lumirubin excretion rate is a function of both the TB level and the irradiance. The relative roles of Z,E-bilirubin and lumirubin can vary significantly. Low irradiance favors the Z,E-bilirubin path; high irradiance favors the lumirubin path. The total excretion rate is lower at lower TB because less light is absorbed by bilirubin and both paths have first-order kinetics.

Other Factors in the Optimization of Phototherapy

Is there a limiting irradiance for phototherapy?

Putting aside limitations caused by the increased heating and oxidative damage rates (vide infra), does phototherapy efficacy saturate at high irradiance?

If the Z,E-bilirubin route were the sole pathway, irradiance sufficient to achieve the pss level of Z,E-bilirubin in a reasonable time would be indicated. Higher irradiance would only result in faster interconversion of configurational isomers, but no change in the phototherapy-mediated excretion rate. Thus, a limiting irradiance on phototherapy efficacy would be expected if only the Z,E-bilirubin pathway operates. The lumirubin pathway has no such restriction and a high irradiance, consistent with safety, would be desired for fastest reduction in TB.

Studies of the irradiance dependence of the 24-hour reduction of TB in near-term infants without hemolytic disease have been made. Tan[45] observed infants of similar GA, BW, Hb level, and initial TB using fluorescent lamps. A more recent study[46] used an LED source ($\lambda_{max} = 460$ nm). However, the infant cohort had large ranges of BW and initial TB, limiting its validity. The study of Tan[45] showed a distinct saturation (leveling off) of the TB decrement rate at high irradiance. The more recent study showed no saturation.

The observation of Tan[45] can be interpreted by comparative rates of bilirubin production and phototherapy-mediated excretion. The average initial TB was 18 mg/dL and the high irradiance average 24-hour TB was 10 mg/dL. The average BW of 2.7 kg corresponds with a net bilirubin production rate (Hb catabolism minus hepatic-mediated excretion) that provides a continuous input into the serum/plasma of about 0.4 mg/dL/h.[47] The rough estimate of the phototherapy excretion rate for 30 μW/cm^2/nm (high end of the irradiance) and a TB of 10 mg/dL (leveling-off point) given in **Table 1** is about the same, at 0.5 mg/dL/h. The leveling-off point simply reflects the balance between phototherapy-mediated excretion and new bilirubin production, and is not an intrinsic limit on irradiance.

Continuous versus cycled (intermittent) phototherapy

If the Z,E-bilirubin pathway for phototherapy dominates, then, with adequate irradiance, the fast increase and saturation of the Z,E-bilirubin level coupled with its slow excretion means that intermittent (cycled) phototherapy could be as effective as continuous phototherapy, because of the continued excretion in the "off" stage of the Z,E-bilirubin produced in the "on" stage. However, because the production of lumirubin is not irradiance limited and lumirubin is excreted at a fairly fast rate, this expectation is counterbalanced by the imposition of the lumirubin pathway. As discussed earlier, the relative contributions of the two pathways depend on both the irradiance and the TB level. The production rate of newly formed bilirubin as well as the durations of the "on" and "off" periods are also key variables, so that the difference in efficacy between continuous and intermittent phototherapy is complex and case specific.

A recent study compared the reduction in TB for infants (GA >34 weeks; no abnormal hemolysis) undergoing continuous or intermittent phototherapy (12 hours off, 12 hours on) at high irradiance.[48] The average starting TB was about 15 mg/dL; there was no correction for Hb level; new bilirubin production rate was assumed to be similar for the two groups. The average decrease in TB for the continuous phototherapy was 1.3 times that for the intermittent phototherapy. That the difference is not a factor of 2 means that there was phototherapy-mediated excretion that extended into the off period as expected. The factor of 1.3 is close to what can be roughly calculated from the relative phototherapy-mediated excretion rates shown in **Table 1** (bottom row). In the study report,[48] it is stated that the intermittent and continuous modes were equally efficacious when viewed as the reduction in TB divided by the dose (irradiance × time), akin to a quantum yield. This view is valid but is deceptive from a clinical view, which might dictate reduction of the TB for an individual infant as quickly as possible.

Several other studies using various on/off ratios and times have shown that cycled phototherapy can be nearly as efficient as continuous phototherapy.[49,50]

Is the production of photoproducts beneficial without excretion?

Because of their water solubility and polarity, it was suggested years ago that Z,E-bilirubin and lumirubin may not effectively cross membranes and the blood-brain barrier and may not be functionally neurotoxic.[11,51] It is further suggested that under aggressive phototherapy the fast (≈1 hour) conversion of 25% or more of TB to these products is significantly neuroprotective even without their excretion, which is a comforting thought.[14,32,51] However, there are no experimental data for the cellular toxicities of Z,E-bilirubin and lumirubin, or for their membrane transport properties. Z,E-bilirubin can thermally reconvert to bilirubin. It is stabilized by binding to albumin (nearly as strong as bilirubin), which may account for its slow excretion. However, separated from albumin, and if it can enter cells, Z,E-bilirubin may convert to bilirubin therein and nothing is gained. Because of practical difficulties, in vitro investigations of the transport and toxic properties of Z,E-bilirubin and lumirubin would be difficult, but should be pursued.

High-risk, very low gestational age, and low body weight infants

Consider a 760-g neonate of 26 weeks' GA with a TB of 8 mg/dL, an Hct of 50%, and no hemolytic disease. With an expected BBC of 14 mg/dL,[23] according to expert recommendation[24] the infant is at risk for bilirubin neurotoxicity and would be prescribed phototherapy. A TB less than or equal to 4 mg/dL would be considered safe. Is there a phototherapy regimen that might reduce the TB to 4 mg/dL in a reasonable time? For this case a net rate of new bilirubin production (heme catabolism minus hepatic excretion) is estimated to be about 0.22 mg/dL.h.[47] According to the rough estimates of **Table 1**, using mLED at 10 μW/cm^2/nm may not be sufficient to keep TB from increasing; 20 μW/cm^2/nm would initially reduce TB by 0.11 mg/dL/h; 30 μW/cm^2/nm would initially reduce TB by 0.21 mg/dL/h. However, because phototherapy becomes progressively slower as the TB is reduced, the TB could only be reduced to about 5 mg/dL unless hepatic excretion improves. If the net rate of new bilirubin production is twice the normal rate because of hemolytic disease, then even an irradiance of 30 μW/cm^2/nm might not be sufficient to maintain the TB at 8 mg/dL. For nonhemolytic cases and an irradiance of 30 μW/cm^2/nm, using cycled phototherapy for 15 minutes on, 45 minutes off (phototherapy-enhanced excretion of 0.22 mg/dL/h) may just be sufficient to keep the TB at 8 mg/dL; 30 minutes on, 30 minutes off (phototherapy-enhanced excretion of 0.28 mg/dL/h) could reduce the TB slowly.

Low GA, low BW infants with low BBC are at risk for bilirubin toxicity at fairly low TB levels and, at the same time, phototherapy is less efficient (measured as reduction of TB per hour) at low TB. This finding is caused by the smaller fraction of phototherapy light that is absorbed by bilirubin at lower TB because of the competition for light absorption by Hb. It is therefore crucial to closely monitor the TB in these infants to ensure that phototherapy is effective. Besides assessment of hemolytic disease, the Hct of these infants should also be considered in deciding whether or not phototherapy can be effective in a timely manner. The estimates of TB decrement rates under phototherapy given earlier are higher by about 20% at an Hct of 40%, and lower by about 15% at an Hct of 60%. There may also be a delay in the expected decrement of TB as bilirubin, which had been residing in extravascular compartments because of the low BBC of the serum, reenters the vasculature.

That the conjecture that Z,E-bilirubin and lumirubin are not effectively neurotoxic may be correct is particularly important for low GA, low BBC infants who are at risk at low TB because aggressive phototherapy can quickly convert up to 30% of the TB to these potentially innocuous products.

A statistically increased mortality in extremely low BW infants under aggressive phototherapy has been observed retrospectively.[52] An increase in heat deposition and/or oxidative stress caused by phototherapy (vide infra) have been invoked as causative.[12]

Oxidative stress

As the wavelength of exposure light is reduced, skin experiences more modes of damage. The association of UVA light (315–400 nm) with skin cancers has necessitated UVA sunscreens. Purported mechanisms for UVA effects on skin extend into the blue light region. In general, these involve formation of free radical and reactive oxygen species (ROS) causing oxidative damage. Increased oxidative stress during phototherapy, especially with aggressive phototherapy, must be considered. Blood levels of flavin-containing moieties are reduced under phototherapy with concomitant increase in blood oxidant/antioxidant status.[53,54] Other sensitizers of ROS, such as adventitious porphyrins, may have a role. Oxyhemoglobin itself is a source of reactive superoxide ions when photolyzed.[55]

A comforting aspect is that bilirubin, even when bound to albumin, is an efficient scavenger of radicals and ROS.[56] However, like other antioxidants, such as vitamin C, low levels of bilirubin may be effective antioxidants, but high levels may support free radical chain processes and exacerbate oxidative damage.

It has been conjectured that blue light–induced oxidative stress may be particularly dangerous for very low birthweight infants under aggressive phototherapy.[52] Two phototherapy parameters might be optimized to reduce oxidative stress: (1) wavelength range, which should be kept as high as possible consonant with effectiveness; and (2) irradiance, which at very high levels might overwhelm protective modes. That is, protection mechanisms may keep up with the formation of oxidants at low, but not at higher, irradiances. This possibility suggests a careful, individualized assessment of the need to quickly reduce TB (aggressive phototherapy) because of the risk for bilirubin toxicity. There should be no hesitation to provide aggressive phototherapy in a crash-cart mode when neurologic symptoms present. Perhaps provision of antioxidants, such as vitamin E, should be reinvestigated.

Optimum phototherapy light source

Light generation technology, the elucidation of skin optics, and progress in understanding of phototherapy processes have converged to provide a strong conclusion for the optimum light source: an array of narrow-band (<25 nm at half height) LEDs with peak wavelength near 475 nm, capable of providing a uniform irradiance greater than or equal to 30 µW/cm²/nm over a 1500-cm² area. Such a source is superior in every important respect: action spectrum overlap, irradiance control, uniformity, stability, safety, and lifetime cost. Narrow-band LED phototherapy units are presently commercially available with peak wavelengths lower than the optimum and are still superior to fluorescent tubes for the reasons given earlier. Manufacturers could easily supply units with the optimum wavelength range.

RESEARCH GAPS

- Availability of facile assays of UB and BBC, useful biomarkers to assess risk of bilirubin toxicity, to augment presently used risk factors.
- An inexpensive standardized irradiance meter tuned to the 460-nm to 490-nm wavelength range.
- Global access to narrow-band LEDs with peak wavelength at 475 nm.
- Elucidation of the cellular toxicity, transport properties, and binding to albumin of Z,E-bilirubin and lumirubin.
- A comprehensive process simulation computer application to guide prescription of infant-specific phototherapy regimens.
- Investigation of the dose and irradiance dependences of oxidative stress markers as well as of heat deposition.

Best practices for effective phototherapy to reduce bilirubin load

What changes in current practice are likely to improve outcomes?

1. Use photons as a drug when prescribing neonatal phototherapy

2. Use of narrow-spectrum blue light (475 nm)

3. Measure irradiance for specific wavelength

4. Use least irradiance dose to achieve an efficient decrease in bilirubin load

5. Consider infants' Hb as a potential barrier for effective bilirubin photodegradation

Clinical Algorithms:

1. Clinical algorithm as proposed by the 2004 American Academy of Pediatrics (AAP) practice guideline[2]

2. Device assessment and use as proposed by the AAP technical report[3]

Strength of the evidence

As listed in the 2010 AAP technical report[3]

Recommendations

Major guidelines for prescription of phototherapy and recommended regimens have become more specific over the years.[24] Based on the attempt discussed earlier to provide a more quantitative pharmacologic view of phototherapy, items of emphasis are offered to augment present guidelines:

- Phototherapy efficacy (defined as the rate of TB reduction) decreases significantly with increased TB and Hct. The efficacy of phototherapy at constant irradiance at a starting TB of 8 mg/dL may only be half of that for a TB of 15 mg/dL. Practitioners must be mindful of this in prescribing a regimen or in deciding whether or not phototherapy is sufficiently timely, especially for low GA infants with low BBCs.
- TB (not transcutaneous bilirubin) should be followed at periodic intervals based on anticipated response to ascertain phototherapy pharmacokinetics, especially for low GA infants.
- A safe-end-point TB level should be determined based on specific parameters to avoid unanticipated rebound hyperbilirubinemia.
- Avoid the use of light outside the range 460 to 490 nm for safest and most efficient phototherapy, and ensure that the irradiance is accurately measured and sufficient.

REFERENCES

1. Ahlfors CE. Criteria for exchange transfusion in jaundiced newborns. Pediatrics 1994;93:488–94.
2. American Academy of Pediatrics. Management of hyperbilirubinemia in the newborn infant 35 or more weeks of gestation. Pediatrics 2004;114:297–316.
3. Bhutani VK, The Committee on Fetus and Newborn. Phototherapy to prevent severe neonatal hyperbilirubinemia in the newborn infant 35 or more weeks of gestation. Pediatrics 2011;128:e1046–52.
4. Hansen TW, Nietsch L, Norman E, et al. Reversibility of acute intermediate phase bilirubin encephalopathy. Acta Paediatr 2009;98:1689–94.
5. Maisels MJ, McDonagh AF. Phototherapy for neonatal jaundice. N Engl J Med 2008;358:920–8.
6. McDonagh AF, Lightner DA. Phototherapy and the photobiology of bilirubin. Semin Liver Dis 1988;8:272–83.
7. Newman TB, Kuzniewicz MW, Liljestrand P, et al. Numbers needed to treat with phototherapy according to American Academy of Pediatrics guidelines. Pediatrics 2009;123:1352–9.
8. Cremer R, Perryman P, Richards DH, et al. Photosensitivity of serum bilirubin. Biochem J 1957;66:60P.
9. Cremer RJ, Perryman PW, Richards DH. Influence of light on the hyperbilirubinaemia of infants. Lancet 1958;1:1094–7.
10. Behrman RE, Hsia DY. Summary of a symposium on phototherapy for hyperbilirubinemia. J Pediatr 1969;75:718–26.
11. McDonagh AF, Lightner DA. "Like a shrivelled blood orange" – bilirubin, jaundice, and phototherapy. Pediatrics 1985;75:443–55.
12. Lamola AA, Bhutani VK, Wong RJ, et al. The effect of hematocrit on the efficacy of phototherapy for neonatal jaundice. Pediatr Res 2013;74:54–60.
13. Bhutani VK, Lamola AA. Mechanistic aspects of phototherapy for neonatal hyperbilirubinemia. In: Polin R, Abman S, Benitz WE, et al, editors. Fetal and neonatal physiology. 5th edition; 2016, in press.
14. Hansen TWR. Neonatal jaundice treatment and management. 2015. Available at: http://medicine.medscape.com/article/974786-treatment. Accessed September 12, 2015.
15. Vreman HJ, Wong RJ, Stevenson DK. Phototherapy: current methods and future directions. Semin Perinatol 2004;28:326–33.
16. Wallenstein MB, Bhutani VK. Jaundice and kernicterus in the moderately preterm infant. Clin Perinatol 2013;40:679–88.
17. Xiong T, Qu Y, Cambier S, et al. The side effects of phototherapy for neonatal jaundice: what do we know? what should we do? Eur J Pediatr 2011;170: 1247–55.
18. Bay State Health. Common NICU medications. 2015. Available at: http://www.baystatehealth.org/services/pediatrics/hospitalization/nicu/support-services/nicu-medications. Accessed September 12, 2015.
19. Watchko JF, Tiribelli C. Bilirubin-induced neurologic damage – mechanisms and management approaches. N Engl J Med 2013;369:2021–30.
20. Ahlfors CE. Predicting bilirubin neurotoxicity in jaundiced newborns. Curr Opin Pediatr 2010;22:129–33.
21. Ahlfors CE, Amin SB, Parker AE. Unbound bilirubin predicts abnormal automated auditory brainstem response in a diverse newborn population. J Perinatol 2009; 29:305–9.

22. Ahlfors CE, Wennberg RP, Ostrow JD, et al. Unbound (free) bilirubin: improving the paradigm for evaluating neonatal jaundice. Clin Chem 2009;55:1288–99.
23. Lamola AA, Bhutani VK, Du L, et al. Neonatal bilirubin binding capacity discerns risk of neurological dysfunction. Pediatr Res 2015;77:334–9.
24. Maisels MJ, Watchko JF, Bhutani VK, et al. An approach to the management of hyperbilirubinemia in the preterm infant less than 35 weeks of gestation. J Perinatol 2012;32:660–4.
25. Jacques SL. Origins of tissue optical properties in the UVA, visible, and NIR regions. In: Afano RR, Fujimoto JG, editors. Advances in optical imaging and photon migration. Washington, DC: Optical Society of America TOPS Proceedings; 1996. p. 374–469.
26. Nielson KP, Zhao L, Stamnes JJ, et al. The optics of human skin: aspects important for human health. In: Bjertness E, editor. Solar radiation and human health. Oslo (Norway): The Norwegian Academy of Science and Letters; 2008. p. 35–46.
27. Jacques SL, Saidi IS, Ladner A, et al. Developing an optical fiber reflectance spectrometer to monitor bilirubinemia in neonates. Proc SPIE 1997;2975:115–24.
28. Ennever JF. Blue light, green light, white light, more light: treatment of neonatal jaundice. Clin Perinatol 1990;17:467–81.
29. Ennever JF, McDonagh AF, Speck WT. Phototherapy for neonatal jaundice: optimal wavelengths of light. J Pediatr 1983;103:295–9.
30. Ebbesen F, Madsen P, Stovring S, et al. Therapeutic effect of turquoise versus blue light with equal irradiance in preterm infants with jaundice. Acta Paediatr 2007;96:837–41.
31. Linfield DT, Lamola AA, Mei E, et al. The effect of hematocrit on in vitro bilirubin photoalteration. Pediatr Res 2015. [Epub ahead of print].
32. Mreihil K, Madsen P, Nakstad B, et al. Early formation of bilirubin isomers during phototherapy for neonatal jaundice: effects of single vs. double fluorescent lamps vs. photodiodes. Pediatr Res 2015;78:56–62.
33. Lightner DA. Bilirubin: Jekyll and Hyde pigment of life. Progress in the chemistry of organic natural products. New York: Springer; 2013.
34. Greene BI, Lamola AA, Shank CV. Picosecond primary photoprocesses of bilirubin bound to human serum albumin. Proc Natl Acad Sci U S A 1981;78:2008–12.
35. Lamola AA, Eisinger J, Blumberg WE, et al. Fluorometric study of the partition of bilirubin among blood components: basis for rapid microassays of bilirubin and bilirubin binding capacity in whole blood. Anal Biochem 1979;100:25–42.
36. Onishi S, Isobe K, Itoh S, et al. Demonstration of a geometric isomer of bilirubin-IX alpha in the serum of a hyperbilirubinaemic newborn infant and the mechanism of jaundice phototherapy. Biochem J 1980;190:533–6.
37. McDonagh AF, Ramonas LM. Jaundice phototherapy: micro flow-cell photometry reveals rapid biliary response of Gunn rats to light. Science 1978;201:829–31.
38. Ennever JF, Knox I, Denne SC, et al. Phototherapy for neonatal jaundice: in vivo clearance of bilirubin photoproducts. Pediatr Res 1985;19:205–8.
39. Lightner DA, McDonagh AF. Molecular mechanisms of phototherapy for neonatal jaundice. Acc Chem Res 1984;17:417–24.
40. Stoll MS, Zenone EA, Ostrow JD, et al. Preparation and properties of bilirubin photoisomers. Biochem J 1979;183:139–46.
41. McDonagh AF, Agati G, Fusi F, et al. Quantum yields for laser photocyclization of bilirubin in the presence of human serum albumin. Dependence of quantum yield on excitation wavelength. Photochem Photobiol 1989;50:305–19.

42. Ennever JF, Costarino AT, Polin RA, et al. Rapid clearance of a structural isomer of bilirubin during phototherapy. J Clin Invest 1987;79:1674–8.
43. Lightner DA. The photoreactivity of bilirubin and related pyrroles. Photochem Photobiol 1977;26:427–36.
44. Lightner DA, Linnane WP 3rd, Ahlfors CE. Bilirubin photooxidation products in the urine of jaundiced neonates receiving phototherapy. Pediatr Res 1984;18:696–700.
45. Tan KL. The nature of the dose-response relationship of phototherapy for neonatal hyperbilirubinemia. J Pediatr 1977;90:448–52.
46. Vandborg PK, Hansen BM, Greisen G, et al. Dose-response relationship of phototherapy for hyperbilirubinemia. Pediatrics 2012;130:e352–7.
47. Maisels MJ, Pathak A, Nelson NM, et al. Endogenous production of carbon monoxide in normal and erythroblastotic newborn infants. J Clin Invest 1971;50:1–8.
48. Sachdeva M, Murki S, Oleti TP, et al. Intermittent versus continuous phototherapy for the treatment of neonatal non-hemolytic moderate hyperbilirubinemia in infants more than 34 weeks of gestational age: a randomized controlled trial. Eur J Pediatr 2015;174:177–81.
49. Vogl TP, Hegyi T, Hiatt IM, et al. Intermediate phototherapy in the treatment of jaundice in the premature infant. J Pediatr 1978;92:627–30.
50. Niknafs P, Mortazavi A, Torabinejad MH, et al. Intermittent versus continuous phototherapy for reducing neonatal hyperbilirubinemia. Iran J Pediatr 2008;18:251–6.
51. Mreihil K, McDonagh AF, Nakstad B, et al. Early isomerization of bilirubin in phototherapy of neonatal jaundice. Pediatr Res 2010;67:656–9.
52. Morris BH, Oh W, Tyson JE, et al. Aggressive vs. conservative phototherapy for infants with extremely low birth weight. N Engl J Med 2008;359:1885–96.
53. Aycicek A, Erel O. Total oxidant/antioxidant status in jaundiced newborns before and after phototherapy. J Pediatr (Rio J) 2007;83:319–22.
54. Gromisch DS, Lopez R, Cole HS, et al. Light (phototherapy)-induced riboflavin deficiency in the neonate. J Pediatr 1977;90:118–22.
55. Balagopalakrishna C, Manoharan PT, Abugo OO, et al. Production of superoxide from hemoglobin-bound oxygen under hypoxic conditions. Biochemistry 1996;35:6393–8.
56. Stocker R, Glazer AN, Ames BN. Antioxidant activity of albumin-bound bilirubin. Proc Natl Acad Sci U S A 1987;84:5918–22.

Biology of Bilirubin Photoisomers

Thor Willy Ruud Hansen, MD, PhD, MHA*

KEYWORDS

- Phototherapy • Jaundice • Neonatal • Bilirubin • Bilirubin photoisomers • Solubility
- Toxicity • Membrane permeability

KEY POINTS

- Phototherapy converts bilirubin to more polar, thus water-soluble, photoisomers. They are excreted in urine and bile, but the excretion profile varies between isomers.
- Physical and biological arguments point to lesser toxicity for bilirubin photoisomers than for native bilirubin-IXα (Z,Z), but in vitro evidence is controversial.
- Given the increased polarity of bilirubin photoisomers, they should be less prone to cross the blood–brain barrier, but no experimental evidence is available to support this hypothesis.
- Phototherapy may not be innocuous in the smallest, most immature infants; whether this is related to aspects of irradiation or the profile of the bilirubin isomer mix, including photo-oxidation products, is unknown.

INTRODUCTION

Jaundice from unconjugated hyperbilirubinemia is arguably the most common reason for diagnostic and therapeutic interventions in newborn infants. Estimates for usage rates in healthy, term infants are mostly in the 2% to 6% rate, depending inter alia on which national guidelines are being used, and also on local practice patterns.[1] In a recent prospective 1-year study of phototherapy use in Norwegian neonatal intensive care units (NICUs), we found that among premature infants at less than 28 weeks gestational age, more than 80% received phototherapy at some point during their NICU stay.[2]

Disclosure: The author has no conflicts of interest, neither financial nor commercial, which are associated with the present work. This work was not funded by any grants, companies, or organizations with interests bearing on the contents of this work.
Division of Paediatric and Adolescent Medicine, Oslo University Hospital, Faculty of Medicine, Institute of Clinical Medicine, University of Oslo, Oslo, Norway
* Nyfødtavdelingen - Rikshospitalet, Barne- og ungdomsklinikken, Oslo Universitetssykehus, Postboks 4950 Nydalen, Oslo 0424, Norway.
E-mail address: t.w.r.hansen@medisin.uio.no

Since the discovery of phototherapy to treat neonatal jaundice,[3] this therapeutic modality is now probably available in all newborn departments as well as maternity wards in the industrialized world. The first phototherapy devices were "home-made" and rather crude.[3] The devices have, in the ensuing 50 years, undergone several stages of advancing technological development. Currently, phototherapy devices using light-emitting diodes seem to be the most widespread, at least in the industrialized part of the world. At the same time, work is ongoing to increase access to phototherapy in low- and middle-income countries by creating much simpler devices that use sunlight and optic filters rather than being dependent on solely electricity and lamps or tubes.[4]

Phototherapy was for a long time regarded as quite harmless, and studies of how it has been used evinced a wide scatter of practical applications.[5,6] This heterogeneity may, in part, be owing to the lack of a solid scientific evidence base, particularly for the smallest and most immature infants. However, there is also an impression that the dispensing and dosing of phototherapy may have been less rigorously controlled than other types of therapy in the NICU. The latter could perhaps be explained on the background of the widespread idea that phototherapy is harmless.

Maisels recalculated the data from the Collaborative Phototherapy Trial,[7,8] and found a relative risk (RR) of death of 1.49 (95% confidence interval [CI], 0.93–2.40) in infants who received phototherapy versus controls.[9] In the original publication, the differences were discounted because they did not reach statistical significance.[8] Recently, Tyson and colleagues[10] published a reanalysis of the data from the National Institute of Child Health and Development Neonatal Research Network study on 'aggressive' versus 'conservative' phototherapy. Using a Bayesian analysis approach, they found that the risk of death was significantly increased (RR, 1.19; 95% CI, 1.01–1.39) in the 501 to 750 g birthweight mechanically ventilated subgroup treated with 'aggressive' phototherapy.

Thus, it is clear that despite more than 50 years of practical use of phototherapy, we still have more to learn. This paper reviews the state of our knowledge regarding the biology of bilirubin photoisomers, the phototherapy products that are thought to be responsible for the effects of this therapeutic modality. The physics and physiology of phototherapy will be only briefly mentioned here for context and for more details (See Lamola AA: A pharmacological view of phototherapy, in this issue).

BILIRUBIN TOXICITY

We treat neonatal hyperbilirubinemia because bilirubin is toxic to the brain. These toxic effects can range from transitory (bilirubin-induced neurologic dysfunction) to the devastating and chronic (kernicterus, chronic bilirubin encephalopathy), and not infrequently also in death.[11] Efforts to discover the 'basic mechanisms' of bilirubin neurotoxicity started more than one-half of a century ago and are ongoing. For details, the interested reader is referred to recent reviews.[11,12] Briefly, bilirubin seems to be toxic in a large number of in vitro systems in which it has been tested. It has been suggested that this could be a false lead, as bilirubin seems to share many of the characteristics of so-called promiscuous inhibitors, compounds that have apparent effects in vitro, but fail to show any such effects when tested in vivo.[13] This author has suggested that such widespread inhibitory effects might also be understood in terms of interference with a basic, common regulatory mechanism such as protein phosphorylation.[12]

The majority of in vitro studies have been performed with bilirubin-IXα (Z,Z), the predominant in vivo isomeric form of bilirubin. The lipophilicity of this isomer enables it to cross membranes, and thus gain entry into cells as well as organs. Important in the latter context is the ability to cross the blood–brain barrier and enter the brain in the absence of any known specific transporter and, similarly in fetal life, to cross the placental barrier from fetus to mother, enabling excretion of bilirubin through the mother's liver.[14] Also, most in vivo studies in intact animal organisms, focusing on bilirubin entry into as well as clearance from the brain, have used bilirubin-IXα (Z,Z), either purified or as the major constituent in a mix of other isomers that share similar lipophilic characteristics.

TYPES OF BILIRUBIN PHOTOPRODUCTS

During phototherapy, bilirubin undergoes partial conversion to stereoisomers. These are more polar than the predominant parent IXα (4Z,15Z) isomer, which needs conjugation to be excreted.[15] Photoisomers are found in serum and, in varying degrees, in bile and urine during phototherapy. The fact that they can be eliminated without need for conjugation in the liver largely accounts for the therapeutic effect of phototherapy as far as lowering total serum/plasma bilirubin (TB) levels. Of the configurational isomers, 4Z,15 E, predominates, (See Lamola AA: A pharmacological view of phototherapy, in this issue) and under NICU phototherapy conditions, has been shown to accumulate to an apparent photostationary level of about 25% of TB.[16,17] The E-isomers can revert to the Z-conformation.

Lumirubin is formed much more slowly than the Z,E-isomers but, because it is more polar, it is excreted much faster, and it does not revert to the Z,Z-conformation (See Lamola AA: A pharmacological view of phototherapy, in this issue). The clearance rate of lumirubin in premature infants has been shown to increase with postconceptional age in parallel with increased creatinine clearance rate.[18] Photooxidation products of bilirubin are not believed to contribute significantly to the therapeutic effect of phototherapy. For more details (See Lamola AA: A pharmacological view of phototherapy, in this issue).

BINDING OF BILIRUBIN ISOMERS

Bilirubin-IXα (Z,Z) is bound to albumin with high affinity at a primary binding site, and a somewhat lower, but still significant affinity at a secondary binding site.[19,20] The binding of bilirubin to albumin is the main factor in protecting cells from toxicity, as only a minute fraction is unbound ("free") and thus able to enter cells (or cross other membranes such as the blood–brain barrier).[21,22] The binding of bilirubin photoisomers has not been studied extensively, but some helpful information is available.

Thus, Lamola and coworkers found that configurationally (Z,E) isomerized bilirubin bound to human serum albumin (HSA) at the primary bilirubin binding site with an affinity only 2 to 3 times lower than that of bilirubin-IXα (Z,Z).[23] The high affinity of photobilirubin for albumin, comparable with that of bilirubin, was believed to support the role of albumin in the stabilization and transport of the isomerized pigment in vivo and to suggest that albumin could also function to sequester photobilirubin, reducing its toxic potential. The high affinity of photobilirubin for albumin predicted that the isomerized pigment should not appear in the fast diazo-reacting ("direct") bilirubin pool, nor should it interfere with nonspectroscopic bilirubin binding tests.

Greene and coworkers[24] concluded that bilirubin remained relatively uninhibited with respect to photoisomerization when bound to HSA. Itoh and Onishi[25] found that (E,Z)-bilirubin photochemically underwent (E,Z)-cyclization, that is, structural photoisomerization, while bound to its high-affinity site on HSA, and was an intermediate in the transformation of (Z,Z)-bilirubin into (E,Z)-cyclobilirubin. In another study, Itoh and coworkers[26] investigated whether bilirubin photoisomers would influence the unbound bilirubin (UB) concentration as estimated by the peroxidase method. They found that the serum polar (Z,E)-bilirubin-IXα concentration increased remarkably during photoirradiation, both in vivo and in vitro, but UB values were not affected at all within the clinically observed range.

Zunszain and colleagues[27] cocrystallized bilirubin with HSA. The crystal structure—determined to 2.42 Å resolution—revealed that the 4Z,15E-bilirubin-IXα isomer was bound to an L-shaped pocket in subdomain IB.[27] Fusidic acid, a competitive displacer of bilirubin from albumin, was found to bind to the same pocket. Unfortunately, it was not possible based on their data to ascertain whether the 4Z,15E-bilirubin bound in the pocket was formed in situ from 4Z,15Z-bilirubin, which had been bound to the same site, or whether it could have been formed by photoisomerization of 4Z,15Z-bilirubin bound to another site, from which 4Z,15 E then migrated to subdomain IB. Whether 4Z,15Z-bilirubin in fact binds to the same site, was not shown by the data, but was suggested by modeling studies.

How bilirubin photoisomers behave with regard to the avidity of their albumin binding will probably require further studies. McDonagh and coworkers[28] performed in vitro studies where they irradiated isomerically pure 4Z,15Z-bilirubin-IXα, while keeping the total amount of bilirubin constant, at the same time ensuring that solutions were not irradiated beyond the initial photostationary state. Free bilirubin in the solutions was then measured with a peroxidase method before and after irradiation. For bilirubin in HSA, conversion of approximately 25% of the 4Z,15Z-isomer to 4Z,15E-bilirubin led to a lesser decrease (<20%) in the apparent UB concentration. However, for bilirubin in serum, conversion of approximately 15% of the 4Z,15Z-isomer to photoisomers resulted in a much greater increase of apparent free bilirubin (approximately 40%). They concluded that UB measurements in a clinical setting need to be interpreted with caution when samples contain photoisomers. Of note, this seems to disagree with the findings of Itoh and colleagues[26] as cited.

Iwase and colleagues[29] compared the specificity of photochemical changes of bilirubin in complex with serum albumin from various species and compared them with HSA. The rates of conversion of the (E,Z)-bilirubin isomer into the structural cyclobilirubin isomer was significantly faster for HSA than for the nonhuman species. The authors speculated that the ability of HSA to facilitate the photochemical change of bilirubin was evolutionarily selected in response to neonatal hyperbilirubinemia in humans.

Bilirubin photoisomers are bound to albumin, possibly to the same site as bilirubin-IXα (Z,Z). Photoisomerization may occur in situ at that binding site, although further confirmation is needed. HSA may facilitate bilirubin photoisomerization compared with albumin from other species. Analyses of UB in infants receiving phototherapy may yield erroneous results.

IN VIVO MODELS OF MEMBRANE PASSAGE

Entry of bilirubin into brain is a sine qua non for its neurotoxic effects, and occurs because bilirubin-IXα (Z,Z) is lipid soluble. Polar molecules, on the other hand, need transporters in the blood–brain barrier to gain access to the neurons. Based on the physical characteristics of the bilirubin photoisomers, it may be hypothesized that these isomers are less able to cross the blood–brain barrier. McDonagh and Lightner[30] suggested almost a quarter of a century ago that the immediate effect of phototherapy—transforming the bilirubin molecule to a presumably less toxic form—might be beneficial and deserved more recognition. Very limited work has been done to follow-up on this suggestion, and it seems not to be discussed in textbooks and guidelines, perhaps because of the dearth of solid data. However, some years ago Maisels and McDonagh[15] raised this issue again and were followed by Hansen.[31,32]

Over the years, several investigators have exposed congenitally jaundiced Gunn rats to phototherapy lights and followed both their TB values as well as brain bilirubin content. In a truly innovative study for its day, Broughton and colleagues[33] studied blue light phototherapy in jaundiced infants and Gunn rats, as well as Wistar rat brain and liver mitochondria incubated with a bilirubin solution exposed to the same light for 32 hours. The in vivo rat study, however, only followed changes in TB that, over a period of 10 days, were shown to be significantly reduced in the light-treated rats versus the controls. Sisson and collaborators[34] exposed Gunn rats to blue light for 21 days and found that it prevented hyperbilirubinemia as well as changes in cerebellar size, ataxia, and (visually assessed) brain discoloration. Other studies, using similar strategies, although with variations in the timing of light exposure as well as methods of brain evaluation, confirmed that the lowering of TB with phototherapy reduced bilirubin entry into brain and/or prevented the changes in brain structure and growth, otherwise typically seen in homozygous Gunn rats.[35,36] With the wisdom of hindsight, the clear limitation of these studies is that they do not really tell us whether photoisomerization in any way influenced bilirubin passage through the blood–brain barrier, except through lowering of TB, which would be expected to lower brain bilirubin.

Cuperus and colleagues[37] created a model with Gunn rats that had either the regular chronic hyperbilirubinemia, or hyperbilirubinemia that was exacerbated by acute hemolysis, and treated them at various intervals with phototherapy, HSA, or phototherapy plus HSA. In the chronic model, adjunct HSA increased the efficacy of phototherapy and decreased plasma free bilirubin and brain bilirubin by 88% and 67%, respectively ($P<.001$). In the acute model, adjunct HSA also increased the efficacy of phototherapy. It decreased plasma UB by 76% ($P<.001$) and completely prevented the hemolysis-induced deposition of bilirubin in the brain. Phototherapy alone failed to prevent the deposition of bilirubin in the brain during acute hemolytic jaundice. Unfortunately, there are limitations in the study design that, in the end, leave the question of bilirubin photoisomers and blood–brain barrier transfer open. Thus, phototherapy was only started 24 hours after the hemolysis-inducing drug was given, and serum bilirubin photoisomers were not measured. Recently, Schreuder and collaborators[38] performed a study in adult Gunn rats in which they compared exchange transfusion, albumin infusion, and phototherapy on TB, UB, and brain bilirubin content. The study design was complex, and because the model was adult Gunn rats, which have had elevated TB levels in their brains for their entire lives, an interpretation of their results for the purposes of our question must be viewed with caution. Also, the authors did not measure bilirubin photoisomers nor did they directly address the crucial question of the ratio between brain and TB levels. Therefore, their results neither support nor disprove a hypothesis of a "brain-sparing" effect of bilirubin photoisomerization.

Thus, there seem to be no studies on record that have used animal models to investigate directly the biology of bilirubin photoisomer transfer from blood to brain. Although protective effects of phototherapy on brain and brain development have been documented, these findings are clearly secondary to lowering of TB, the primary effect of phototherapy, and do not speak to the issue of bilirubin photoisomers and their increased polarity relative to blood–brain barrier passage.

However, another natural model of photoisomer membrane passage is worth considering. Gajdos and coworkers[39] describe a patient who, having been under life-long phototherapy treatment for Crigler-Najjar syndrome type 1, had enjoyed completely normal neurodevelopment. At the age of 28 years, her first pregnancy began while her TB concentration was 400 μmol/L (23.5 mg/dL) with a bilirubin/albumin molar ratio of 0.52. Phototherapy was intensified, to which were added biweekly infusions of albumin at 1 g/kg. This combination maintained TB between 230 and 280 μmol/L (13.5 and 16.5 mg/dL), and the bilirubin/albumin ratio remained at less than 0.45 for the duration of the pregnancy. At birth, the mother's TB was 242 μmol/L, and the infant's was 247 μmol/L at 1 hour of age. TB in the umbilical artery and the umbilical vein were both 222 μmol/L. All of the TB was unconjugated.

Although the results of analyses of TB in general should not be overinterpreted, given the recognition that analytical precision is far from perfect, some reflections may be permissible. Thus, the fetal values of TB, as reflected in the umbilical vessel values, were certainly not higher, and possibly slightly lower than the mother's. Whether fetal-to-maternal transfer of bilirubin is solely a passive process (involving diffusion), requiring a fetal-to-maternal concentration gradient, or may involve active transport, is not entirely clear.[14] In some studies, the fetal-to-maternal gradient has been estimated to be between 1:5 and 1:10.[40,41] Rosenthal[40] found that the TB concentration in the umbilical artery was twice that of the umbilical vein, indicating that bilirubin was cleared from fetal blood when crossing the placenta. Although Gajdos and coworkers[39] did perform high-performance liquid chromatography analyses of the bilirubin content in both maternal and fetal samples, these were focused on bilirubin conjugates and not on photoisomers. However, a speculation seems possible: assuming the mother's TB had reached a photostationary balance of about 25% of the Z,E-isomer and 75% of the Z,Z-isomer, as seems achievable in neonatal phototherapy,[16,17] then there was a real fetal-to-maternal concentration gradient of the Z,Z-isomer, possibly explaining why the fetal TB was not higher than the maternal, as might have been expected. Although in no way constituting proof of the hypothesis concerning bilirubin photoisomers and membrane passage, at least these observations may be compatible with the hypothesis.

IN VITRO TOXICITY STUDIES

A number of in vitro studies have examined the effects of bilirubin photoproducts. The results, alas, are far from conclusive. In some studies, there seems to be evidence of increased cellular toxicity when cells are exposed to phototherapy in the presence of bilirubin.[42–44] However, given the study conditions the results may not be relevant for our question. Mainly, irradiation conditions were such that it seems likely that significant photooxidation occurred, leading to oxidative cell damage.[44] Other studies seem to support a hypothesis of less toxicity for the bilirubin photoproducts.[33,45–48] However, the interpretation of these results should be guarded because the experimental conditions, both as far as light flux and isomer composition, are variable and in several papers not well, or not at all, defined.

It is notable that Broughton and associates,[33] as early as in 1965 argued that "the toxicity of bilirubin has been attributed to its fat solubility, and it seems probable that the water-soluble products would, therefore, be less toxic, and also more easily excreted," Fat solubility versus polarity are, theoretically, strongly linked to ability to cross cell and tissue membranes and, therefore, quite possibly to toxic mechanisms. Based on their experiments, Broughton and coworkers concluded that "there is no evidence that the products of light treatment are toxic."

With the benefit of what has been learned in the 5 decades since the Broughton publication,[33] this conclusion cannot be sustained on the basis of the methods they used. Thus, the stability of the bilirubin solution they used is questionable, and the bilirubin concentration in their control solution was extremely high, opening to criticism as far as 'nonphysiologic' experimental conditions.[49] The contents of the bilirubin solution after 32 hours of irradiation could not be analyzed for photoisomers because these were not known. Given the experimental conditions, the irradiated solution likely contained significant amounts of photooxidation products. However, if this were the case, the lack of toxicity reported by the authors is surprising. This makes the unknown length of exposure of the mitochondria to the solutions a final stumbling block in our attempts to interpret these data.

Silberberg and coworkers[50] exposed myelinating rat cerebellar cultures for 24 hours to either 30 mg/dL (510 μmol/L) bilirubin (B:A ratio 1.7:1), or to the same solution of bilirubin that had been exposed to blue light of unknown irradiance for 6 hours, and in which remaining diazo-positive material corresponded with 14 mg/dL bilirubin (240 μmol; B:A ratio 0.8:1). Controls were exposed to incubation solution without bilirubin added. In cultures exposed to irradiated bilirubin solution neurons were not damaged. However, nonirradiated bilirubin solutions produced characteristic and severe damage of the neurons. Like the study by Broughton and coworkers,[33] this study was also interpreted to show that photodegradation products of bilirubin are less toxic than the native compound.[50] But the problems as far as interpreting the significance of the findings are really the same as for Broughton's study. We cannot know what these photodegradation products were, nor in what concentrations they occurred. It still seems likely that photooxidation products may have been a significant constituent. Also, one would have expected that the diazo-positive products, which remained after irradiation, if they truly represented bilirubin-IXα (Z,Z), would have caused cell toxicity. Thus, we probably cannot accept this study as proof that bilirubin photoisomers lack toxicity.

An important contribution to the understanding of the impact of experimental conditions on in vitro studies of bilirubin photoisomer toxicity came from Sideris and coworkers.[43] They studied DNA replication, frequency of sister chromatid exchanges, and survival in cultured Chinese hamster cells exposed to light in the blue spectral band between 420 and 500 nm. The results showed that light of this band length is largely responsible for DNA breaks, sister chromatid exchanges, and lethality induced by fluorescent light. Their data suggest that in vitro studies of bilirubin photoisomer toxicity should be interpreted with caution if exposure to bilirubin solution and light occurred concurrently.

Rosenstein and coworkers[44] exposed normal human fibroblasts to light at 420 to 490 nm with exogenously added 1 to 100 μg/mL of bilirubin. Other cells were incubated in the dark with bilirubin solutions that had been preirradiated. Control cells were irradiated in solutions without added bilirubin. This study seems to be compatible with the suggestion that the increased toxicity observed in a number of studies using high and prolonged doses of light in the presence of bilirubin may be owing more to oxidation products than to bilirubin or its isomers.

Several valuable studies have come from Christensen's group at the Norwegian Radiation Protection Authority. In an early study, Chinese V79 hamster cells were irradiated at 20 W/m^2 for varying periods of time, at a bilirubin concentration of 10 mg/dL (170 μmol/L).[45] Cell survival evinced a bell-shaped curve, with almost complete survival at around 30 minutes (estimated from Figure 1 in the original paper), and proceeding toward complete cell death when irradiation times exceeded 90 minutes (again estimated from Figure 1 in the original paper). The authors' interpretation was that increased survival at lower exposures was owing to formation of bilirubin photoisomers, whereas increased death at higher light doses was likely owing to formation of photooxidation products. The survival curve was similar whether the cells were incubated in bilirubin solution that had been preexposed to light, or whether cells were present during light exposure. Unfortunately, the phototherapy products were not characterized, only assumed. The finding that the toxic effects were not observed in the presence of human serum, but were reproducible in calf serum, is of particular interest, because the rates of conversion of the (E,Z)-bilirubin isomer into the structural cyclobilirubin isomer were previously shown to be significantly higher in the presence of HSA than in albumin from nonhuman species.[29]

In their next study, Christensen and coworkers[51] used the human glioblastoma cell line TMG-1 and exposed the cells to blue or green light in the absence or presence of bilirubin. Irradiance for the blue light was 64 W/m^2 and for the green light 32 W/m^2. Blue light induced single-strand breaks in the DNA of cells in culture, even in the absence of bilirubin. At high and clinically relevant bilirubin concentrations, toxic effects were relatively similar under both blue and green lights, whereas at lesser concentrations there was less toxic effect of green light as expected from the absorption spectrum of bilirubin.

Christensen and Kinn[52] then went on to study how bilirubin photoisomerization might be influenced by the presence of cells. Cultured cells from 1 human and 1 murine cell line were incubated with bilirubin by different methods that allowed bilirubin to be bound to cells. The cells, as well as bilirubin bound to human serum in the absence of cells, were irradiated with visible light of different wavelengths. No photoisomers were found in samples of irradiated cell-containing solutions, whereas the types and amounts of photoisomers that were expected from the literature were found in samples of irradiated bilirubin/albumin mixtures. It seems difficult to reconcile the data from cell cultures in this study with the prior study by Christensen and colleagues,[45] where it is argued that cell toxicity is ameliorated by bilirubin photoisomers, whether cells are exposed to preirradiated bilirubin solution or irradiation, occurs in the presence of both cells and bilirubin.

A later study by Christensen and colleagues[46] may, on a closer inspection of their data and figures, yield some insight into the relative toxicities of photooxidation products versus lumirubins, Z,E- or E,Z-isomers. Thus, a possible interpretation seems to be that photooxidation products played a main role in the cytotoxic effects observed in murine lymphoma cells exposed to blue light and 160 μmol/L of bilirubin. Cell survival was stable in the presence of HSA for 2 hours, although photooxidation products may be inferred to constitute about 50% of the incubation mixture at this time. The amount of lumirubin was not quantitated, but Iwase and colleagues[29] suggested that lumirubin formation would be expected to proceed much more rapidly in the presence of HSA, possibly explaining the high cell survival. However, please note that this interpretation may be speculative, as several details are not reported in the paper, and have been inferred from figures and tables.

In another study by Roll and Christensen,[48] mouse lymphoma cells were again used as a model. The results suggest that green light contributed to more formation of lumirubin than blue light, and that the photoproducts from green light irradiation were less cytotoxic than those resulting from blue light irradiation. However, it is difficult to interpret these results. The suitability of the cell model must be questioned, because the data seemed to show that a solution of native Z,Z-bilirubin had limited cytotoxicity, a finding contrary to most other studies of bilirubin cell toxicity. Second, the formation of presumably toxic photooxidation products was considerable, thus making it difficult to assess which products of irradiated bilirubin should account for what effects. Similar limitations seem to apply regarding the interpretation of a subsequent study by Roll, using the same cell model.[47]

More recent data from Calligaris and colleagues[53] show reduced toxicity of light-irradiated bilirubin in cell cultures, although the interpretation of this finding is limited by lacking documentation of what the actual photoproducts were. Furthermore, the change in toxicity paralleled the change in UB in the solution, and thus may not be directly related to the photoproducts per se. In this context, it should be noted that phototherapy seems to reduce serum UB more than TB, reducing the UB:TB ratio,[54] and consequently the driving force for bilirubin to enter the cells.

No studies seem to be on record as having studied cellular uptake of bilirubin photoisomers.

CLINICAL IMPLICATIONS

Bilirubin photoisomers are formed within minutes of starting effective phototherapy.[16,17] Clinical evidence supports the role of rapidly instituted and intensive phototherapy in preventing and even reversing acute bilirubin encephalopathy.[55–57] The putative role of photoisomerization in such "brain rescue" remains to be proven. Although the experimental evidence with regard to the biology of bilirubin photoisomers is incomplete and apparently contradictory, the risk–benefit ratio in applying crash-cart phototherapy to infants with very high TB levels and evidence of ongoing neurotoxicity or threat of same, is strongly in favor of "flipping the switch" as soon as possible. This approach is illustrated in the clinical algorithm (**Fig. 1**).[58]

Although measuring bilirubin photoisomers is currently not practical in day-to-day NICU management of jaundiced infants, practicing neonatologists should be aware of the physics and physiology of these isomers and apply our current understanding of their role to management of neonatal hyperbilirubinemia.

The site of action of phototherapy is most likely in the capillaries of the skin.[59] A key concept, which all neonatologists need to keep in mind, is spectral power — the product of irradiance and the size of the irradiated area. There may not be a saturation point for spectral power or irradiance in phototherapy as far as effects on TB are concerned.[60] Whether this applies to photoisomers has not been studied. The practical implication in the NICU must be to make every effort to maximize spectral power. Phototherapy lights in the turquoise-to-green spectrum may be more effective than blue for lowering TB.[61] Whether this would play any role in crash-cart phototherapy remains to be studied.

SUMMARY

Since the serendipitous discovery of phototherapy as an important therapeutic approach for neonatal jaundice, the physics and physiology of bilirubin photoisomerization have been extensively studied as reviewed by Lamola AA (See Lamola AA: A pharmacological view of phototherapy, in this issue). Unfortunately, our understanding of the biology of bilirubin photoisomers seems to be lagging behind. In a recent publication, Mreihil and coworkers[16] argued as follows:

With respect to bilirubin toxicity, there are, a priori, three possibilities: the photoisomer has similar toxicity to the "natural" isomer; the photoisomer is more toxic; or the photoisomer is less toxic. Of these, the first is unlikely because of the different structures and physicochemical properties of the two forms and the need for pigment to enter the brain to cause toxicity. The second possibility also seems unlikely because countless phototherapy treatments over the last half-century seem never to have caused or exacerbated CNS toxicity. This leaves the third possibility; the most likely in view of the much lower lipophilicity of the photoisomer compared with the 4Z,15Z-isomer, which would be expected to make it less prone to cross the blood–brain barrier and enter the brain.

Thus, the theoretic arguments are chemically and physiologically coherent. The reports of apparent reversibility of acute intermediate-to-advanced stage bilirubin

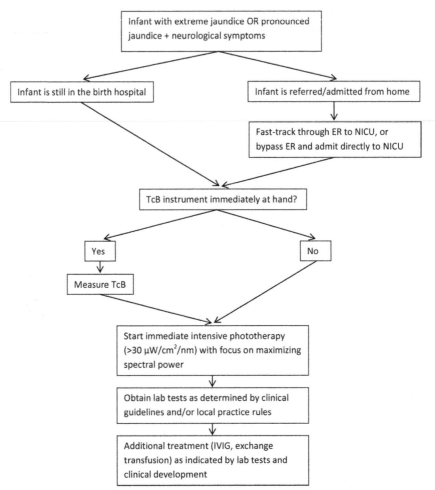

Fig. 1. Clinical algorithm. ER, emergency room; IVIG, intravenous immunoglobulin; NICU, neonatal intensive care unit; TcB, transcutaneous bilirubin.

encephalopathy with timely aggressive therapy may also be interpreted to support this hypothesis.[55–57] Unfortunately, as clearly shown in this review, experimental models to test this hypothesis have been hard to devise. Thus, significant methodologic problems are connected with the solubility and stability of bilirubin and its isomers in aqueous solutions as well as the responses of cells to irradiation. In an animal model, any study designed to examine acute effects would require the ability to achieve and maintain a balanced composition of bilirubin isomers in an infusate, recognizing that only a proportion of the bilirubin in this solution would be photoisomers, and the majority would still be bilirubin-IXα (Z,Z), with its well-documented ability to cross the blood–brain barrier. However, owing to the increasing concern about the purported resurgence of kernicterus in industrialized countries, its persistence in low- and middle-income countries, and the need to adequately test the role of phototherapy in the crash-cart approach to extreme neonatal hyperbilirubinemia, it seems more necessary than ever to attempt to answer the questions discussed in this review.

Best practices

What is current practice?

Infants with risk factors for jaundice, or presenting with visually apparent jaundice, are screened with transcutaneous bilirubin or a blood test for TB.

Therapeutic intervention consists primarily of phototherapy.

Institution of therapy is commonly delayed until the results of these test(s) is/are available and have been assessed.

Phototherapy is deployed using fluorescent tubes or light-emitting diodes, typically in the blue color range, with the light source situated above or beneath the infants, or both concurrently.

The effect of therapy is measured with tests for TB.

In infants admitted from home, delays in admission procedures or testing are not infrequent, leading to delayed initiation of treatment.

What changes in current practice are likely to improve outcomes?

Fast tracking of jaundiced infants through emergency rooms, or admitting directly to NICUs will reduce delays (see **Fig. 1**).

Infants with pronounced/extreme hyperbilirubinemia, particularly if also presenting with any kind of neurologic symptomatology, should have intensive phototherapy ($>30 \ \mu W/cm^2/nm$) started immediately without waiting for test results (of any kind).

Maximizing spectral power (irradiance multiplied by the size of the irradiated area) will contribute to rapid formation of bilirubin photoisomers ($\sim 10\%$ after 15 minutes, $\sim 25\%$ after 2 hours). Bilirubin isomers are more polar (water soluble) than native bilirubin-IXα (Z,Z), and may be less likely to enter the brain.

Summary statement

This article reviews the evidence regarding the biology of bilirubin photoisomers. Although the evidence from in vitro studies is not clearcut, the physics and physiology of photoisomers suggest that an approach, which ensures rapid formation of such isomers is likely to be "brain sparing" in extreme neonatal hyperbilirubinemia.

REFERENCES

1. Darling EK, Ramsay T, Sprague AE, et al. Universal bilirubin screening and health care utilization. Pediatrics 2014;134:e1017–24.

2. Mreihil K, Nakstad B, Stensvold HJ, et al. Phototherapy treatment (Px) for neonatal jaundice (NJ) in Norwegian NICUs - a prospective national survey. San Diego (CA): Pediatric Academic Societies; 2015. Publication 1579.582.

3. Cremer RJ, Perryman PW, Richards DH. Influence of light on the hyperbilirubinaemia of infants. Lancet 1958;1:1094–7.

4. Slusher TM, Olusanya BO, Vreman HJ, et al. A randomized trial of phototherapy with filtered sunlight in African neonates. N Engl J Med 2015;373:1115–24.

5. Hansen TW. Therapeutic practices in neonatal jaundice: an international survey. Clin Pediatr (Phila) 1996;35:309–16.

6. Gartner LM, Herrarias CT, Sebring RH. Practice patterns in neonatal hyperbilirubinemia. Pediatrics 1998;101:25–31.

7. Brown AK, Kim MH, Wu PYK, et al. Efficacy of phototherapy in prevention and management of neonatal hyperbilirubinemia. Pediatrics 1985;75:393–400.

8. Lipsitz PJ, Gartner LM, Bryla DA. Neonatal and infant mortality in relation to phototherapy. Pediatrics 1985;75:422–6.

9. Maisels MJ. Neonatal jaundice. In: Sinclair JC, Bracken MB, editors. Effective care of the newborn infant. Oxford (England): Oxford University Press; 1992. p. 507–61.

10. Tyson JE, Pedroza C, Langer J, et al. Does aggressive phototherapy increase mortality while decreasing profound impairment among the smallest and sickest newborns? J Perinatol 2012;32:677–84.

11. Watchko JF, Tiribelli C. Bilirubin-induced neurologic damage — mechanisms and management approaches. N Engl J Med 2013;369:2021–30.

12. Hansen TWR. Mechanisms of bilirubin-induced brain injury [Chapter 122]. In: Polin RA, Fox WW, Abman SH, editors. Fetal and neonatal physiology. 4th edition. Philadelphia: Elsevier Saunders; 2011. p. 1295–306.

13. McDonagh AF. Controversies in bilirubin biochemistry and their clinical relevance. Semin Fetal Neonatal Med 2010;15:141–7.

14. Hansen TWR, Bratlid D. Physiology of neonatal unconjugated hyperbilirubinemia [Chapter 5]. In: Stevenson DK, Maisels MJ, Watchko JF, editors. Care of the jaundiced neonate. New York: McGraw-Hill; 2012. p. 65–96.

15. Maisels MJ, McDonagh AF. Phototherapy for neonatal jaundice. N Engl J Med 2008;358:920–8.

16. Mreihil K, McDonagh AF, Nakstad B, et al. Early isomerization of bilirubin in phototherapy of neonatal jaundice. Pediatr Res 2010;67:656–9.

17. Mreihil K, Madsen P, Nakstad B, et al. Formation of bilirubin photoisomers during single and double fluorescent vs photodiode phototherapy. Pediatr Res 2015;78: 56–62.

18. Knox I, Ennever JF, Speck WT. Urinary excretion of an isomer of bilirubin during phototherapy. Pediatr Res 1985;19:198–201.

19. Brodersen R. Binding of bilirubin to albumin. Crit Rev Clin Lab Sci 1980;11: 305–99.

20. Brodersen R. Bilirubin. Solubility and interaction with albumin and phospholipids. J Biol Chem 1979;254:2364–9.

21. Jacobsen J, Wennberg RP. Determination of unbound bilirubin in the serum of newborns. Clin Chem 1974;20:783–9.

22. Cashore WJ. Free bilirubin concentrations and bilirubin-binding affinity in term and preterm infants. J Pediatr 1980;96:521–7.

23. Lamola AA, Flores J, Blumberg WE. Binding of photobilirubin to human serum albumin - estimate of the affinity constant. Eur J Biochem 1983;132:165–9.

24. Greene BI, Lamola AA, Shank CV. Picosecond primary photoprocesses of bilirubin bound to human serum albumin. Proc Natl Acad Sci U S A 1981;78: 2008–12.

25. Itoh S, Onishi S. Kinetic study of the photochemical changes of (*ZZ*)-bilirubin IX alpha bound to human serum albumin. Demonstration of (*EZ*)-bilirubin IX alpha as an intermediate in photochemical changes from (*ZZ*)-bilirubin IX alpha to (*EZ*)-cyclobilirubin IX alpha. Biochem J 1985;226:251–8.

26. Itoh S, Yamakawa T, Onishi S, et al. The effect of bilirubin photoisomers on unbound-bilirubin concentrations estimated by the peroxidase method. Biochem J 1986;239:417–21.

27. Zunszain PA, Ghuman J, McDonagh AF, et al. Crystallographic analysis of human serum albumin complexed with 4*z*,15*e*-bilirubin-IXα. J Mol Biol 2008;381: 394–406.

28. McDonagh AF, Vreman HJ, Wong RJ, et al. Photoisomers: obfuscating factors in clinical peroxidase measurements of unbound bilirubin? Pediatrics 2009;123: 67–76.

29. Iwase T, Kusaka T, Itoh S. (EZ)-Cyclobilirubin formation from bilirubin in complex with serum albumin derived from various species. J Photochem Photobiol B 2010; 98:138–43.

30. McDonagh AF, Lightner DA. Like a shrivelled blood orange. Bilirubin, jaundice and phototherapy. Pediatrics 1985;75:443–55.

31. Hansen TW. Phototherapy for neonatal jaundice - therapeutic effects on more than one level? Semin Perinatol 2010;34:231–4.

32. Hansen TW. The role of phototherapy in the crash-cart approach to extreme neonatal jaundice. Semin Perinatol 2011;35:171–4.

33. Broughton PG, Rossiter EJ, Warren CB, et al. Effect of blue light on hyperbilirubinaemia. Arch Dis Child 1965;40:666–71.

34. Sisson TR, Goldberg S, Slaven B. The effect of visible light on the Gunn rat: convulsive threshold, bilirubin concentration, and brain color. Pediatr Res 1974; 8:647–51.

35. Kashiwamata S, Aono S, Semba RK. Characteristic changes of cerebellar proteins associated with cerebellar hypoplasia in jaundiced Gunn rats and the prevention of these by phototherapy. Experientia 1980;36:1143–4.

36. Keino H, Kashiwamata S. Critical period of bilirubin-induced cerebellar hypoplasia in a new Sprague-Dawley strain of jaundiced Gunn rats. Neurosci Res 1989;6: 209–15.

37. Cuperus FJ, Schreuder AB, van Imhoff DE, et al. Beyond plasma bilirubin: the effects of phototherapy and albumin on brain bilirubin levels in Gunn rats. J Hepatol 2013;58:134–40.

38. Schreuder AB, Vanikova J, Vitek L, et al. Optimizing exchange transfusion for severe unconjugated hyperbilirubinemia: studies in the Gunn rat. PLoS One 2013;8: e77179.

39. Gajdos V, Petit F, Trioche P, et al. Successful pregnancy in a Crigler-Najjar type I patient treated by phototherapy and semimonthly albumin infusions. Gastroenterology 2006;131:921–4.

40. Rosenthal P. Human placental bilirubin metabolism. Pediatr Res 1990;27:223A.

41. Monte MJ, Rodriguez-Bravo T, Macias RI, et al. Relationship between bile acid transport gradients and transport across the fetal-facing plasma membrane of the human trophoblast. Pediatr Res 1995;38:156–63.

42. Christensen T, Kinn G, Granli T, et al. Cells, bilirubin and light: formation of bilirubin photoproducts and cellular damage at defined wavelengths. Acta Paediatr 1994;83:7–12.

43. Sideris EG, Papageorgiou GC, Charalampous SC, et al. A spectrum response study on single strand DNA breaks, sister chromatide exchanges, and lethality induced by phototherapy lights. Pediatr Res 1981;5:1019–23.

44. Rosenstein BS, Ducore JM, Cummings SW. The mechanism of bilirubin-photosensitized DNA strand breakage in human cells exposed to phototherapy light. Mutat Res 1983;112:397–406.

45. Christensen T, Støttum A, Brunborg G, et al. Unwanted side effect and optimization of phototherapy. Light Biol Med 1988;1:153–9.

46. Christensen T, Roll EB, Jaworska A, et al. Bilirubin- and light-induced cell death in a murine lymphoma cell line. J Photochem Photobiol B 2000;58:170–4.

47. Roll EB. Bilirubin-induced cell death during continuous and intermittent phototherapy and in the dark. Acta Paediatr 2005;94:1437–42.

48. Roll EB, Christensen T. Formation of photoproducts and cytotoxicity of bilirubin irradiated with turquoise and blue phototherapy light. Acta Paediatr 2005;94: 1448–54.

49. Ostrow JD, Tiribelli C. New concepts in bilirubin neurotoxicity and the need for studies at clinically relevant bilirubin concentrations. J Hepatol 2001;34:467–70.
50. Silberberg DH, Johnson L, Schutta H, et al. Effects of photodegradation products of bilirubin on myelinating cerebellum cultures. J Pediatr 1970;77:613–8.
51. Christensen T, Reitan JB, Kinn G. Single-strand breaks in the DNA of human cells exposed to visible light from phototherapy lamps in the presence and absence of bilirubin. J Photochem Photobiol B 1990;7:337–46.
52. Christensen T, Kinn G. Bilirubin bound to cells does not form photoisomers. Acta Paediatr 1993;82:22–5.
53. Calligaris SD, Bellarosa C, Giraudi P, et al. Cytotoxicity is predicted by unbound and not total bilirubin concentration. Pediatr Res 2007;62:576–80.
54. Nakamura H, Lee Y, Uetani Y, et al. Effects of phototherapy on serum unbound bilirubin in icteric newborn infants. Biol Neonate 1981;39:295–9.
55. Harris MC, Bernbaum JC, Polin JR, et al. Developmental follow-up of breastfed term and near-term infants with marked hyperbilirubinemia. Pediatrics 2001; 107:1075–80.
56. Johnson L, Bhutani VK, Karp K, et al. Clinical report from the pilot USA kernicterus registry (1992 to 2004). J Perinatol 2009;29(Suppl 1):S25–45.
57. Hansen TW, Nietsch L, Norman E, et al. Apparent reversibility of acute intermediate phase bilirubin encephalopathy. Acta Paediatr 2009;98:1689–94.
58. Smitherman H, Stark AR, Bhutani VK. Early recognition of neonatal hyperbilirubinemia and its emergent management. Semin Fetal Neonatal Med 2006;11: 214–24.
59. Donneborg ML, Knudsen KB, Ebbesen F. Effect of infants' position on serum bilirubin level during conventional phototherapy. Acta Paediatr 2010;99:1131–4.
60. Vandborg PK, Hansen DM, Greisen G, et al. Dose-response relationship of phototherapy for hyperbilirubinemia. Pediatrics 2012;130:e352.
61. Ebbesen F, Madsen P, Støvring S, et al. Therapeutic effect of turquoise versus blue light with equal irradiance in preterm infants with jaundice. Acta Paediatr 2007;96:837–41.

Phototherapy and the Risk of Photo-Oxidative Injury in Extremely Low Birth Weight Infants

CrossMark

David K. Stevenson, MD[a], Ronald J. Wong, BS[a,*],
Cody C. Arnold, MD, MSc, MPH[b], Claudia Pedroza, PhD[b],
Jon E. Tyson, MD, MPH[b]

KEYWORDS

- Bilirubin • Reactive oxygen species • Photosensitivity
- Bilirubin-induced neurologic dysfunction

KEY POINTS

- The safety and efficacy of phototherapy have not been specifically tested as a drug in extremely low birth weight (ELBW) infants.
- The vulnerability of an ELBW infant to light-induced oxidative damage must be considered.
- An infant's hematocrit (Hct) may affect the efficacy of phototherapy, especially in ELBW infants; a lower Hct may allow for more penetration of light.

INTRODUCTION

Phototherapy has been used to treat newborns with jaundice for over half a century with the presumption that it is safe and effective for all infants. In fact, this presumption may not be true for all infants, especially the smallest and most immature. The safety and efficacy of phototherapy have never really been questioned or adequately tested in the latter, yet clinical applications of phototherapy have been further refined as its mechanisms of action have been better understood and alternative light sources have become available. This article addresses what is known about the possible risks of photo-oxidative injury in extremely low birth weight (ELBW) infants.

Author Disclosure: None of the authors have financial relationships and conflicts of interest to disclose relevant to this article.
[a] Division of Neonatal and Developmental Medicine, Department of Pediatrics, Stanford University School of Medicine, 750 Welch Road, Suite #315, Stanford, CA 94305, USA;
[b] Department of Pediatrics, University of Texas Health Science Center at Houston, 6431 Fannin Street MSB 3.020, Houston, TX 77030, USA
* Corresponding author. Department of Pediatrics, Stanford University School of Medicine, 300 Pasteur Drive, Room S230, Stanford, CA 94305.
E-mail address: rjwong@stanford.edu

Clin Perinatol 43 (2016) 291–295
http://dx.doi.org/10.1016/j.clp.2016.01.005
0095-5108/16/$ – see front matter © 2016 Elsevier Inc. All rights reserved.

PHOTOTHERAPY USE IN EXTREMELY LOW BIRTH WEIGHT INFANTS

Until recently, improvements in the efficacy of phototherapy have been mainly from the practice of increasing the radiant flux emitted by a phototherapy device to an infant's skin surface. This is accomplished by: (1) using a light source that can emit more energy (irradiance, $\mu W/cm^2/nm$) at the wavelengths shown to photodegrade bilirubin; (2) moving a particular light source closer to the baby; or (3) exposing more of an infant's body surface area to the light. Historically, wide-spectrum white light (most commonly emitted by fluorescent tubes) has been used, but unfortunately, infants were being exposed to extraneous light wavelengths, which were ineffective and possibly dangerous. Since the introduction of narrow-band light-emitting diode (LED) light sources, the wavelength applied during phototherapy is optimized to degrade the bilirubin molecule,[1–3] with minimal or no extraneous light. Most LED devices emit blue light in a narrow range (± 10 nm) with a peak emission at approximately 450 nm. Actually, bilirubin has peak absorption around 478 nm and slightly more effective lights (in terms of wavelength emitted) are technically possible.[2] Another factor that can affect efficacy is how much light is available to interact with bilirubin. A molecule, such as hemoglobin, has an absorption spectrum that substantially overlaps with that of bilirubin, and hence can compete with bilirubin for light. Therefore, in infants with lower hematocrits (Hcts), more "light" (at least that which can be absorbed by bilirubin) is available to interact with bilirubin.[4,5]

VULNERABILITY OF EXTREMELY LOW BIRTH WEIGHT INFANTS

All of these preceding observations should be especially considered in the application of phototherapy to ELBW infants, who are immature with limited antioxidant defenses. Notably, the only large, randomized trial of phototherapy involving infants was conducted in the 1970s and reported in 1985 by Brown and colleagues.[6] They reported that phototherapy (at that time typically fluorescent white tubes were used) was shown to reduce the use of exchange transfusion, an important finding that changed clinical practice dramatically. However, the study was insufficiently powered to draw any conclusions about one vexing observation, that is, the risk of death relative to control subjects, especially for the lowest birth weight stratum: relative risk was 1.49 (95% confidence interval, 0.93–2.40) for infants with birth weight less than 1000 g.[6] This was observed even at a time when light sources emitted much lower irradiances and presumably with limited exposure to damaging wavelengths. Nonetheless, the trend toward a higher mortality in the light-exposed preterm infants less than 2500 g was still apparent (relative risk, 1.32; 95% confidence interval, 0.96–1.82).[7] Since then, the dose of phototherapy light has increased with improvements in light source technology, the placement of lights in closer proximity to the infant, or a deliberate effort to increase an infant's exposed body surface area. Also, what has changed over the years is that the infants being treated with phototherapy have become steadily smaller with thinner and more translucent skin. In fact, the overgeneralization of the efficacy and safety of phototherapy to its application in ELBW infants is a prime example of what Silverman had advised avoiding.[8] These smaller infants also have lower Hcts (thus less light-absorbing hemoglobin), allowing more of the light to interact not only with bilirubin, but also with molecules in many other tissues inside the body.[4,5] One of the most worrisome tissues in this regard is the brain, because an infant's head represents a large proportion of the total surface area compared with that of an adult. If one places a flashlight on an ELBW infant's head, the potential vulnerability of the infant is quickly revealed. The recent National Institute of Child Health and Development Neonatal Research Network paper comparing aggressive versus conservative phototherapy for ELBW infants[9] is an echo of the 1970s collaborative study,[6] and suggests a tradeoff between reducing the risk for bilirubin-induced neurologic dysfunction and increasing the risk for death, a formidable dilemma for doctors and parents.[9,10]

Recently, Arnold and colleagues[11] reviewed the evidence for clinical trials regarding efficacy and safety, making the case for prudence in practice and for the need for more randomized controlled trials involving phototherapy in ELBW infants. The two large phototherapy trials, conducted several decades apart, serve as the basis for their cautionary conclusions and recommendations. They make the point that bilirubin is not the only molecule likely to be affected by the application of light, especially to a translucent ELBW infant, who also may be stressed in other ways. Many side effects of light, in particular broad-spectrum visible light, have been reported,[12,13] but most have not been shown to have adverse or severe clinical consequences. However, one effect, the generation of free radicals and reactive oxygen species from photo-oxidation, is particularly worrisome.[12] In fact, there is no dispute about the occurrence of such photo-oxidative reactions with phototherapy as a side effect of its main mechanism of action. The latter is photoisomerization of bilirubin to form various E,Z-isomers, which are water-soluble and can be excreted in urine and bile without conjugation (and presumed to be nontoxic), and to produce lumirubin, a structural isomer of bilirubin that is excreted in bile.[14] However, we have observed that the application of white and blue fluorescent tube lights to newborn rats can result in rapid and dramatic photo-oxidation reactions as evidenced by increases in in vivo carbon monoxide (CO) production, mainly from the skin, but presumably also from internal tissues reached by the light.[15] CO can be produced via several mechanisms, such as photo-oxidation and the peroxidation of membrane lipids and other organic compounds.[12,15,16] Although blue LED light was less photo-oxidizing, it still resulted in a measurable increase in CO production.[15]

Another factor that has not been explored systematically is whether the presence of other photosensitizers, such as riboflavin (either endogenous or given through parenteral nutrition), in the circulation of ELBW infants might further increase their vulnerability to light exposure.[15,17] Besides hemolysis, other oxidative risks could result from riboflavin photosensitization. At higher bilirubin levels, bilirubin itself is photosensitizing, playing a different role from its usual antioxidant one at lower levels.[16,18] This irony is true of other antioxidant molecules, depending on their concentration and the local biochemical context of the oxidant stress.

Unfortunately clinicians have not considered light as a drug and associated dose-dependent effects. Their tools, photometers, for monitoring light "dosing" have been truncated to the specifications of certain light sources or to only parts of the spectral range of light emitted by a particular light source. A clinician can thus be misled and even blinded to the full irradiance or dose of light emitted by the device. Because humans are immersed in light during most of our waking hours, we do not notice it—we live in it; but ambient light and phototherapy conditions, especially in neonatal intensive care units, are highly variable and potentially can affect the health of infants, and even under certain conditions, may cause injury.[19]

Thus, to properly apply phototherapy, its dosing, duration of exposure, wavelength of light used, and emitted irradiance are critical. Recent work by Lamola and colleagues[4,5] suggests that even an infant's Hct level should be considered when making decisions about dosing.

SUMMARY/DISCUSSION

The current state of knowledge requires that clinicians reserve judgment on the safety of phototherapy for ELBW infants until further randomized controlled trials are conducted. In the meantime, although treatment of hyperbilirubinemia is still required to protect ELBW infants from bilirubin-induced neurologic dysfunction, perhaps even at lower levels of bilirubin than previously appreciated because of compromised bilirubin-binding capacity in ELBW infants,[20] especially in the first several days after birth, caution with the application of light is warranted—another echo of the past.[21] Even shielding of the head might be considered, although the head represents a disproportionately large surface area in the ELBW infant. To reiterate Arnold and colleagues,[11] minimally effective irradiance using a narrow-spectrum LED light source emitting light in the range of maximum bilirubin absorption following a cycled phototherapy regimen should be considered. In the end, a nonphototherapy solution for treating hyperbilirubinemia in ELBW infants may still be the best option.[22,23]

Best practices

What is current practice?

- Neonatologists should consider use blue LED light phototherapy in the wavelength range of 450 to 475 nm with minimum irradiance of at least 8 to 10 $\mu W/cm^2/nm$ to most effectively reduce total serum/plasma bilirubin (TB) while minimizing any risks of phototherapy and track the response in serial TB levels.

- For infants with excessive hyperbilirubinemia, intensive phototherapy is applied at an irradiance of about 30 $\mu W/cm^2/nm$ while considering the use of exchange transfusion.

- The effectiveness of phototherapy in reducing TB depends on duration of exposure, wavelength of light used, and emitted irradiance.

What changes in current practice are likely to improve outcome?

- Clinical trials are needed to determine the optimal "dosing" of phototherapy for infants according to their gestational age, birth weight, TB, clinical risk factors, and Hct to minimize potential light-induced cell damage and the risk of bilirubin-induced neurotoxicity.

- The use of "cycled" phototherapy should be evaluated in a large trial as an option for use in treating ELBW infants.

- The use of compounds to inhibit bilirubin production (eg, enteral zinc protoporphyrin) should be evaluated in a large trial as an option for use in ELBW infants.

Summary Statement

A re-evaluation of the parameters used to deliver phototherapy to ELBW infants will reduce the possible risks of photo-oxidative injury in these small translucent infants.

REFERENCES

1. Seidman DS, Moise J, Ergaz Z, et al. A new blue light-emitting phototherapy device: a prospective randomized controlled study. J Pediatr 2000;136:771–4.
2. Vreman HJ, Wong RJ, Stevenson DK. Phototherapy: current methods and future directions. Semin Perinatol 2004;28:326–33.
3. Vreman HJ, Wong RJ, Stevenson DK, et al. Light-emitting diodes: a novel light source for phototherapy. Pediatr Res 1998;44:804–9.
4. Lamola AA, Bhutani VK, Wong RJ, et al. The effect of hematocrit on the efficacy of phototherapy for neonatal jaundice. Pediatr Res 2013;74:54–60.

5. Linfield DT, Lamola AA, Mei E, et al. The effect of hematocrit on in vitro bilirubin photoalteration. Pediatr Res 2015. http://dx.doi.org/10.1038/pr.2015.240.

6. Brown AK, Kim MH, Wu PY, et al. Efficacy of phototherapy in prevention and management of neonatal hyperbilirubinemia. Pediatrics 1985;75:393–400.

7. Maisels MJ. Neonatal jaundice. In: Sinclair JC, Bracken MB, editors. Effective care of the newborn infant. New York: Oxford University Press; 1992. p. 507–61.

8. Silverman WA. Ambitious overgeneralisation. Paediatr Perinat Epidemiol 2002;16: 288–9.

9. Morris BH, Oh W, Tyson JE, et al. Aggressive vs. conservative phototherapy for infants with extremely low birth weight. N Engl J Med 2008;359:1885–96.

10. Oh W, Stevenson DK, Tyson JE, et al. Influence of clinical status on the association between plasma total and unbound bilirubin and death or adverse neurodevelopmental outcomes in extremely low birth weight infants. Acta Paediatr 2010; 99:673–8.

11. Arnold C, Pedroza C, Tyson JE. Phototherapy in ELBW newborns. Does it work? Is it safe? The evidence from randomized clinical trials. Semin Perinatol 2014;38: 452–64.

12. Magidson V, Khodjakov A. Circumventing photodamage in live-cell microscopy. Methods Cell Biol 2013;114:545–60.

13. Wu PY, Wong WH, Hodgman JE, et al. Changes in blood flow in the skin and muscle with phototherapy. Pediatr Res 1974;8:257–62.

14. McDonagh AF, Lightner DA. Phototherapy and the photobiology of bilirubin. Semin Liver Dis 1988;8:272–83.

15. Vreman HJ, Knauer Y, Wong RJ, et al. Dermal carbon monoxide excretion in neonatal rats during light exposure. Pediatr Res 2009;66:66–9.

16. Vreman HJ, Wong RJ, Sanesi CA, et al. Simultaneous production of carbon monoxide and thiobarbituric acid reactive substances in rat tissue preparations by an iron-ascorbate system. Can J Physiol Pharmacol 1998;76:1057–65.

17. Sisson TR. Photodegradation of riboflavin in neonates. Fed Proc 1987;46:1883–5.

18. Stocker R, Yamamoto Y, McDonagh AF, et al. Bilirubin is an antioxidant of possible physiological importance. Science 1987;235:1043–6.

19. Landry RJ, Scheidt PC, Hammond RW. Ambient light and phototherapy conditions of eight neonatal care units: a summary report. Pediatrics 1985;75:434–6.

20. Lamola AA, Bhutani VK, Du L, et al. Neonatal bilirubin binding capacity discerns risk of neurological dysfunction. Pediatr Res 2015;77:334–9.

21. Preliminary report of the committee on phototherapy in the newborn infant. J Pediatr 1974;84:135–43.

22. Schulz S, Wong RJ, Vreman HJ, et al. Metalloporphyrins: an update. Front Pharmacol 2012;3:68.

23. Stevenson DK, Rodgers PA, Vreman HJ. The use of metalloporphyrins for the chemoprevention of neonatal jaundice. Am J Dis Child 1989;143:353–6.

Bilirubin-Induced Neurotoxicity in the Preterm Neonate

Jon F. Watchko, MD

KEYWORDS

- Kernicterus • Excitotoxicity • Low-bilirubin kernicterus • Auditory neuropathy
- Cerebellum • Hypoalbuminemia

KEY POINTS

- Bilirubin-induced neuronal injury likely reflects the adverse nature of hazardous unbound unconjugated bilirubin on plasma membranes and resultant excitotoxicity, neuroinflammation, oxidative stress, and perturbed cell cycle kinetics, including cell cycle arrest.
- Hazardous hyperbilirubinemia leading to acute bilirubin encephalopathy is increasingly recognized to adversely impact neural respiratory drive and manifest clinically as recurrent symptomatic central, mixed, and obstructive apnea events.
- Low-bilirubin kernicterus is a rare, but refractory cause of bilirubin-induced neurotoxicity in preterm neonates. Although low-bilirubin kernicterus is multifactorial in its pathogenesis, marked hypoalbuminemia is often a prominent clinical feature.

INTRODUCTION

The potential for bilirubin-induced neurotoxicity in the premature neonate (<37 weeks gestational age [GA]) remains a clinical concern. In addition to classic kernicterus, the preterm infant is at risk for auditory predominant chronic bilirubin encephalopathy (CBE) and low-bilirubin kernicterus.[1,2] Others suggest that bilirubin neurotoxicity in preterm neonates may be associated with less severe neurodevelopmental disabilities, a putative condition termed subtle kernicterus or bilirubin-induced neurologic dysfunction (BIND).[1] These conditions and postulated mechanisms of bilirubin-induced central nervous system (CNS) injury are highlighted in this review.

Disclosure Statement: Dr J.F. Watchko reports serving as a consultant in legal cases related to neonatal jaundice. No other potential conflict of interest relevant to this article was reported.
Support: The Mario Lemieux Foundation and The 25 Club of Magee-Womens Hospital.
Division of Newborn Medicine, Department of Pediatrics, Magee-Womens Hospital, Children's Hospital of Pittsburgh, Magee-Womens Research Institute, University of Pittsburgh School of Medicine, 300 Halket Street, Pittsburgh, PA 15213, USA
E-mail address: jwatchko@mail.magee.edu

NEUROPATHOLOGY OF KERNICTERUS

The neuropathology of bilirubin-induced brain damage is (i) remarkably similar across preterm and term neonates, and murine animal models; (ii) distinct from hypoxic-ischemic neonatal CNS injury; and (iii) notable in sparing the neocortex.[1,3] Classic kernicterus at postmortem in the preterm neonate is characterized by both (i) intense yellow staining of neurons in selected brainstem nuclear clusters and (ii) histopathologic evidence of neuronal damage in these stained regions. However, bilirubin staining in the *absence* of characteristic microscopic evidence of neuronal injury does not constitute kernicterus.[3] Brainstem regions typically affected in kernicterus include the following: the (i) globus pallidus; (ii) subthalamic nuclei; (iii) metabolic sector of the hippocampus; (iv) oculomotor nuclei; (v) ventral cochlear nuclei; (vi) Purkinje cells of the cerebellar cortex; and (vii) cerebellar dentate nuclei.[3]

NEUROIMAGING OF KERNICTERUS

MRI of the infant with kernicterus mirrors the distinct regional nature of bilirubin-induced neuropathology demonstrating abnormal bilateral, symmetric, high-intensity signals in the globus pallidus and subthalamic nuclei and on occasion the internal capsule and thalamus (**Fig. 1**).[4,5] Chronic bilateral, symmetrically increased T2-signal (or T2-FLAIR [fluid attenuated inversion recovery] signal) in the globus pallidus and subthalamic nuclei of an infant with a history of hyperbilirubinemia remains the neuroimaging hallmark of kernicterus. These structural MRI findings are equally apparent in affected preterm[6,7] and term neonates.

The subcortical regions affected in CBE are interconnected with each other as well as other cortical and subcortical brain regions via numerous white matter tracts (eg, cortico-ponto-cerebello-thalamo-cortical pathway, cortico-striato-thalamo-cortical pathways).[5] It is therefore expected that *advanced* MRI techniques, including diffusion-weighted imaging, apparent diffusion coefficient mapping, and diffusion tensor imaging with tractography, will shed insight into the abnormalities of structural and functional neural connectivity that underlie the long-term disability in infants and

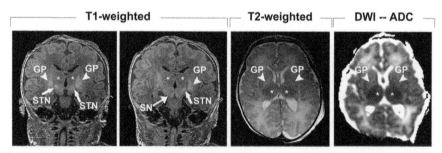

Fig. 1. Conventional MRI performed on postnatal day 5 in an infant who went on to develop CBE. Coronal T1-weighted, axial T2-weighted, and axial-apparent diffusion coefficient (ADC) images are shown. Increased T1-signal is readily apparent in the globus pallidus (GP) and subthalamic nucleus (STN), with more subtle evidence of increased T1-signal in the substantia nigra and hippocampus (not labeled). There is also subtle increased T2-signal in the GP. Remarkably, the ADC images did not demonstrate any restricted diffusion in the GP; however, there was subtle evidence of restricted diffusion in the ventrolateral nucleus of the thalamus, posterior limb of the internal capsule, and the hippocampus (not pictured). *, thalamus; DWI-ADC, diffusion-weighted image-apparent diffusion coefficient. (*From* Wisnowski JL, Panigrahy A, Painter M, et al. Magnetic resonance imaging of bilirubin encephalopathy: current limitations and future promise. Semin Perinatol 2014;38:424; with permission.)

children with CBE.[5] Use of magnetic resonance spectroscopy (MRS) of affected regions of interest may also shed new insights into the pathobiology of bilirubin-induced brain injury.[5]

MOLECULAR AND CELLULAR MECHANISMS OF BILIRUBIN NEUROTOXICITY

The complex cascades of molecular and cellular events that underlie bilirubin-induced neurotoxicity remain incompletely understood, but involve regional and cell-specific responses.[8] **Fig. 2** highlights the multiple reported effects of bilirubin on neurons and glia cells.[8] Which of these effects constitute the "core" processes or molecular triggers that ultimately lead to bilirubin neurotoxicity is unclear.[8–12] Nevertheless, the pathogenesis of bilirubin-induced neuronal cell injury likely reflects the adverse effects of hazardous unbound unconjugated bilirubin (UB) concentrations on plasma, mitochondrial, and/or endoplasmic reticulum membranes (**Fig. 3**).[8,12] These membrane perturbations, in turn, precipitate untoward cellular events that culminate in increased intracellular calcium concentrations (iCa^{2+}). Downstream events triggered by increased iCa^{2+} may include the activation of proteolytic enzymes, apoptosis, necrosis, as well as abnormalities of cell cycle progression, including cell cycle arrest.

Bilirubin and Membranes

The main isomer of bilirubin in humans is bilirubin-IXα (Z,Z), an amphipathic molecule, but one that has a high affinity for membrane lipids.[13,14] Several studies suggest that membranes are the primary or initiating targets of bilirubin toxicity (reviewed in Ref. [12]). However, there is surprisingly little information regarding the actual nature of bilirubin-membrane complexes under physiologic conditions and clinically relevant UB concentrations, nor information on why not all cell types or tissues bind bilirubin with equal affinity.[15] Zucker and colleagues[14] showed that the amphipathic nature of bilirubin facilitates interaction with phospholipid bilayers, localizing to the polar region near the membrane-water interface. Disruption of phospholipid asymmetry, inhibition of membrane-bound ATPases, lipid peroxidation, and other adverse sequelae may ensue.[16] Analogous bilirubin-induced adverse changes in mitochondrial membranes have also been reported.[17] Future studies further characterizing bilirubin-phospholipid membrane complexes and their localization are warranted.[15] In this regard, Ly and colleagues[18] recently shared preliminary findings that lipid raft microdomains may be a target of bilirubin toxicity and amenable to therapeutic intervention.

Excitotoxicity

Excitotoxicity has been proposed to contribute to bilirubin-induced CNS injury on the basis of compelling in vitro, in vivo, and MRI studies. Glutamate, the primary excitatory neurotransmitter in the CNS, and the N-methyl-D-aspartate (NMDA) glutamate receptor subtype are important in the pathogenesis of neonatal neuronal injury.[19] Once NMDA channels are open, downstream events of excitotoxicity become manifest, including (i) an early rapid glutamate receptor activation that leads to increased intracellular Na^+ and Cl^- and resultant cell swelling; followed by (ii) a delayed phase of Ca^{2+} influx and Ca^{2+} release from intracellular stores leading to activation of Ca^{2+}-dependent enzymes that activate apoptosis and/or necrosis.[20] Bilirubin-induced excitotoxicity may develop from a sustained period of mitochondrial energy failure with resultant neuronal depolarization and passive opening of NMDA glutamate channels.[19,21,22] Indeed, Novelli and colleagues[22] report that reduced intracellular energy levels are prerequisites for excitotoxicity; glutamate alone is necessary, but not sufficient.

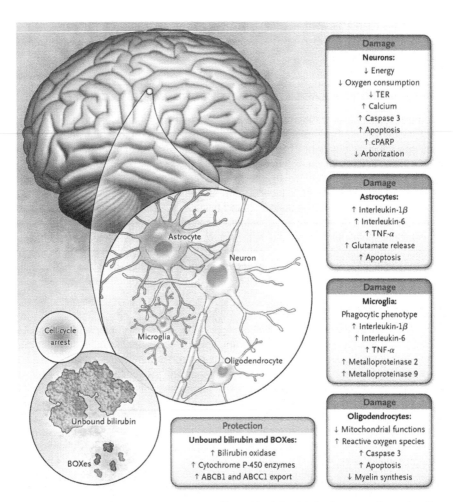

Fig. 2. Cell types and metabolic processes affected by bilirubin in the CNS. The main effects of bilirubin on neurons are decreased oxygen consumption and increased release of calcium and caspase 3, resulting in apoptosis. There is also decreased dendritic and axonal arborization. A similar pattern is observed in oligodendrocytes with increased apoptosis, impairment of the redox state (oxidative stress), and reduced synthesis of myelin. Microglia react to toxic injury associated with bilirubin by increased release of proinflammatory cytokines and metalloproteinase activity as cells manifest a phagocytic phenotype. A similar proinflammatory pattern is observed in astrocytes with enhanced release of glutamate and apoptosis. At the same time, cells may reduce the intracellular concentration of bilirubin either by extruding the pigment through the ATP-binding cassette transporters or by increasing the formation of the less toxic products through bilirubin oxidation products (BOXes) and/or cytochrome P-450 enzymes (1a1 and 1a2 in particular). These responses are protective, whereas all others result in cell damage; this suggests that once the intracellular concentration of bilirubin exceeds a toxic threshold (still to be defined), the polymorphic metabolic cascade leading to neurotoxicity ensues. cPARP, cleaved poly(adenosine diphosphate-ribose) polymerase; TER, transcellular resistance. (*From* Watchko JF, Tiribelli C. Bilirubin-induced neurologic damage—mechanism and management approaches. N Engl J Med 2013;369:2025; with permission from Massachusetts Medical Society.)

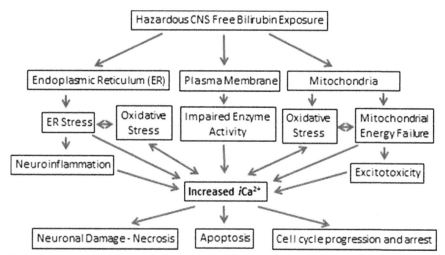

Fig. 3. Schematic of several hypothesized pathophysiological mechanisms in bilirubin-induced neuronal injury. Hazardous UB exposure in the CNS exerts direct effects at the level of the plasma membrane, mitochondria, and/or endoplasmic reticulum (ER), leading to ER stress, oxidative stress, impaired enzyme activity, and mitochondrial energy failure, culminating in neuroinflammation, excitotoxicity, and increased iCa^{2+}. If CNS UB exposure is of sufficient degree and/or duration than irreversible neuronal damage, that is, necrosis, and/or cell cycle arrest may ensue. (*Adapted from* Watchko JF. Kernicterus and the molecular mechanisms of bilirubin-induced CNS injury in newborns. Neuromolecular Med 2006;8(4):518; with permission.)

Excitotoxicity and mitochondrial energy failure suggest a possible explanation for the regional nature of bilirubin-induced CNS damage.[19,21] Neurons of the neonatal globus pallidus show a high resting (baseline) level of neuronal activity[21] and a high neuronal glutamate receptor density.[23] The former makes the region relatively more susceptible to subacute energy failure, whereas the latter would accentuate excitotoxicity injury. Consistent with this hypothesis are (i) evidence of excitotoxicity injury in the Gunn rat model of kernicterus[24]; and (ii) the reported cerebral metabolic signature on proton MRS of an elevated glutamate and glutamine:creatine ratio during acute severe hyperbilirubinemia.[25]

Neuroinflammation

Conditions associated with severe systemic inflammation, including sepsis, necrotizing enterocolitis, and the fetal inflammatory response syndrome (chorioamnionitis with funisitis) are each reported to potentiate bilirubin neurotoxicity.[2] This potentiating effect may be greater in less mature cells and in preterm neonates[26–28] and modulated by endoplasmic reticulum stress, the activation of nuclear factor-κB, and the unfolded protein response.[29] Hazardous levels of UB alone are also immunostimulatory and induce acute and chronic microglial activation in vivo, upregulate pro-inflammatory gene expression, and trigger the cellular (microglia and astrocyte) release of tumor necrosis factor-α (TNF-α), interleukin (IL)-1β, and IL-6 to produce a proinflammatory milieu.[2,8–10,26] Proinflammatory cytokines in turn enhance bilirubin-induced neuronal apoptosis and necrosis in monoculture.[9,10,26] These bilirubin-induced neuroinflammatory responses might contribute to neurologic damage.

Recent studies, however, suggest a more complex dynamic, including evidence that early bilirubin-induced proinflammatory responses can paradoxically be neuroprotective.[30,31] The toll-like receptor 2 (TLR2) signaling pathway appears to be linked to hyperbilirubinemia-induced activation of microglia, astrocytes, resultant reactive gliosis, upregulation of TNF-α, IL-1β, IL-6 gene expression, and pronounced neuroinflammation in vivo.[30] Deletion of TLR2 in mice blocks the induction of these inflammatory cytokine genes yet is associated with increased cerebellar apoptosis and higher neonatal death rates.[30] These data suggest that TLR2 signaling and early neuroinflammation are neuroprotective.[30] Consistent with this complex dynamic, astrocytes in a coculture with neurons can protect or aggravate bilirubin-induced neurotoxicity depending on the duration of the cell-cell communication (preconditioning) and bilirubin exposure.[31]

In addition, chronic neuroinflammation is now recognized as an important risk factor for CNS injury in preterm neonates. In this regard, chronic bilirubin-induced neuroinflammation (microglial activation) is reported in the Gunn rat model of kernicterus and appears in association with abnormal brain development.[32,33] The possibility that bilirubin-induced CNS injury may extend beyond the initial insult via chronic inflammation is intriguing and suggests there may be a therapeutic window following acute bilirubin encephalopathy (ABE). This possibility merits clarification as does the study of possible neuroprotective intervention(s) targeted to inflammatory responses within the complex "yin and yang" of neuroinflammation.[34]

Oxidative Stress

Signs of oxidative stress are consistently associated with hazardous levels of bilirubin in vitro and in vivo and therefore feature prominently in many models of bilirubin-induced neurotoxicity. Nevertheless, it remains unclear whether bilirubin-induced oxidative stress is causally linked to bilirubin neurotoxicity. For example, although several equipotent antioxidants (minocycline; 12S-hydroxy-1,12-pyrazolinominocycline [PMIN]; taurourosdexoycholic acid) consistently and robustly reduce lipid peroxidation (4-hydroxynonenal) during ABE in the Gunn rat model of kernicterus, only minocycline prevents neurotoxicity.[35] This finding suggests that lipid peroxidation inhibition alone is not sufficient to prevent ABE and that the neuroprotective efficacy of minocycline involves action(s) independent of or in addition to its antioxidant effects. It also suggests that caution is warranted in inferring causal linkage between a bilirubin-induced effect and bilirubin neurotoxicity.

Bilirubin and Intracellular Calcium Homeostasis

Regardless of triggering mechanisms, it does appear that increased iCa^{2+} levels are critical to the development of bilirubin-induced cell injury (see **Fig. 3**).[10,12,16] Consistent with this assertion, PMIN, a noncalcium chelating derivative of minocycline, is not neuroprotective against ABE in the Gunn rat model of kernicterus, whereas calcium-chelating minocycline is.[35] Hazardous UB itself may further elevate iCa^{2+} levels by adversely impairing iCa^{2+} buffering via calmodulin-dependent protein kinase II,[36] calbindin, and parvalbumin.[37,38] Once developed, high iCa^{2+} levels via second messenger pathways may activate proteases, lipases, and endonucleases and trigger the generation of free radicals, a series of events that culminate in cell death via either apoptosis or necrosis.[10,12,16]

Perturbed Cell Cycle Kinetics, Cell Cycle Arrest, Altered Neurogenesis

In addition to cell death, hazardous bilirubin levels may adversely impact cell cycle kinetics. In this regard, the most consistent feature of bilirubin-induced neurotoxicity in both the Gunn rat and the *UGT1* knockout mouse models is cerebellar hypoplasia. Recent investigations suggest this may largely be a consequence of perturbed cell cycle progression and apoptosis.[39] More specifically, Gunn rat cerebella show increased cell cycle arrest in late G0/G1, decreased cyclin D1, cyclin A/A1, cyclin-dependent kinase 2, and an increase in cyclin E, which augments apoptosis.[39] Bilirubin-impaired cell cycle progression, cell cycle arrest in G0/G1, and resultant marked reduction in number of proliferating cells are also observed in vitro (**Fig. 4**) and related to bilirubin concentration and exposure duration.[40] These cytostatic effects may be mediated by a variety of neuropeptides, neurotrophins, or growth factors, including among others fibroblast growth factor 1, insulin growth factor 1, sonic hedgehog (SHH), brain-derived neurotrophic factor, glial-derived neurotrophic factor, and neurotrophic factor 3. A preliminary study suggests that the SHH-smoothened signaling axis is not involved.[41] Cerebellar injury to Purkinje cells, the dentate nucleus, and cerebellar roof nuclei is a consistent feature of kernicterus neuropathology in human neonates.

Central Nervous System Immaturity

Few in vitro studies have explored developmental aspects of bilirubin effects on the CNS. Falcao and colleagues[42] studying rat cortical neurons at different duration of days in vitro (DIV) observed that "immature" neurons, that is, those with shorter DIV,

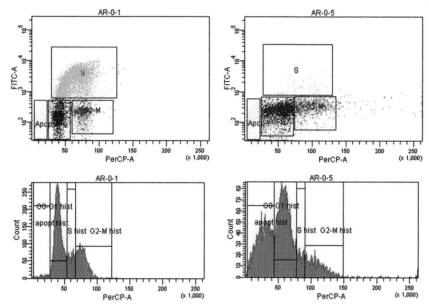

Fig. 4. Cell cycle kinetics determined by flow cytometry during hazardous UB exposure. Representative fluorescence activated cell sorting (FACS) dot plots (*top panels*) show marked changes in the distribution of human promyelocytic leukemia (HL-60) cells using fluorescein isothiocyanate (FITC) -labeled BrdU and correlative histograms (*bottom panels*) during 500-nM UB exposures of 24-hour duration (*right panels*) compared with control HL-60 cells (*left panels*). Notably, there is a marked increase in the number of cells in the G0/G1 phase, a decrease in the number of cells in the S phase, and an increase in the number of cells in apoptosis, consistent with bilirubin-induced cell cycle arrest in G0/G. AR-0-5, an internal shorthand for the parent HL-60 cell line used in this study at 500 nm bilirubin exposure; AR-0-1, parent cell HL-60 cell line under control conditions; PerCP-A, Peridinin-chlorophyll protein-A (the reagent used in the flow cytometry). (*From* Daood MJ, Azzuqa A, Watchko JF. Bilirubin-induced cytostasis, G0/G1 cell cycle arrest, and apoptosis as function of increasing concentration and duration of exposure in vitro. E-PAS 2014;4525.1.)

were more vulnerable to bilirubin-induced injury as manifest by apoptosis and reduction in neurite growth and branching. Notably, the Gunn rat and *UGT1* knockout mouse in vivo kernicterus models are representative of the preterm rather than the term neonate. CNS development in these murine species between birth and postnatal day 10 mirrors that seen in preterm human neonates between 24 and 38 weeks GA.[43] Thus, they offer a powerful experimental approach to study the effects of bilirubin on early postnatal preterm CNS injury.

Future Basic Research Efforts

Hazardous UB concentrations adversely affect many subcellular compartments and biochemical pathways. Despite the considerable efforts of numerous investigators in the field, a robust unifying hypothesis or consensus model of bilirubin neurotoxicity has yet to be firmly established: one that is parsimonious and consistent with the classic features of kernicterus neuropathology, neuroimaging, and neurologic outcomes. Basic research endeavors must strive to more fully integrate insights obtained in vitro (cell lines, coculture systems, and slice preparations) with those obtained in vivo (murine models) and ultimately those observed in human neonates (neuropathology and neuroimaging) to distinguish causal relationships from epiphenomenon. Investigators must also come full circle in their efforts to ensure that insights gained in basic research are relevant to human biology and ultimately translatable to the clinical arena.

Clinical Manifestations of Bilirubin-Induced Central Nervous System Injury in the Preterm Neonate

Acute bilirubin encephalopathy

ABE describes an altered neurologic state induced by hazardous hyperbilirubinemia during the first days of postnatal life characterized by a constellation of abnormal clinical signs typically progressive in their severity. In mature infants, the initial phase of ABE is characterized by stupor (lethargy), hypotonia, and poor sucking. These nonspecific signs are seen in numerous clinical contexts, but, in a hyperbilirubinemic infant, should raise the possibility of early ABE. Clinical signs of intermediate to advanced stages of ABE are increasingly more specific to bilirubin-induced neurotoxicity and herald a marked increased risk for permanent damage. These signs include hypertonia often manifested by retrocollis and opisthotonos, fever, and high-pitched cry. Apnea and inability to feed may ensue. Any infant with signs of intermediate to advanced ABE (hypertonia, arching, retrocollis, opisthotonos, fever, high-pitched cry) merits an immediate exchange transfusion in an attempt to avert CBE.[44,45]

Preterm neonates less frequently show these classic abnormal neuromotor signs, making it difficult to recognize ABE in the some preterm neonates. Recurrent apnea and desaturations may be the only clinical manifestations of ABE in preterm infants during the neonatal period, if any appear at all. Hazardous hyperbilirubinemia is increasingly recognized to adversely impact neural respiratory drive and lead to central, mixed, and obstructive apnea events.[46] Symptomatic apneic events, sometimes manifest as "cyanotic attacks," are reported in premature infants.[46,47] Some suggest disordered control of breathing is a "distinctive picture" of ABE in preterm infants or at least a prominent clinical feature.[46,47] Therefore, recurrent symptomatic apneic events in a jaundiced neonate should prompt a total serum bilirubin (TB) measurement and evaluation for ABE.[46,48] Such events result from bilirubin-induced brainstem injury and blunted ventilatory responses to Pa_{CO_2} and or Pa_{O_2}.[46]

Chronic bilirubin encephalopathy

In contrast to ABE, CBE defines the permanent clinical sequelae of bilirubin toxicity that become evident in the first year of life and is synonymous with the term kernicterus.[1,45] The American Academy of Pediatrics recommends the term kernicterus be reserved for the chronic and permanent neurologic sequelae of bilirubin toxicity.[45] In classic kernicterus, these include the extrapyramidal movement disorders of dystonia and/or choreoathetosis, hearing loss due to auditory neuropathy spectrum disorder (ANSD), and the eye movement abnormality of paresis of upward gaze.[1] Dental enamel hypoplasia may also be seen in association with these neurologic findings. Classic kernicterus is well described in preterm neonates and possibly the most frequent manifestation of bilirubin-induced brain damage in this patient population.

Auditory-predominant kernicterus

The retrocochlear structures of the auditory system (brainstem auditory nuclei, inferior colliculi, and VIII cranial nerve) are vulnerable to bilirubin neurotoxicity. Auditory-predominant kernicterus can result, a subtype of CBE in which ANSD are the primary sequelae[1]; abnormalities in motor control and muscle tone, if present, are subtle.[1] Shapiro[1] suggests that auditory predominant kernicterus is more common in preterm neonates. Hearing screens in the neonatal intensive care unit must therefore include an auditory brainstem-evoked response in addition to otoacoustic emissions in order to detect affected infants with bilirubin-induced injury to the auditory pathway.

Low-Bilirubin Kernicterus

Low-bilirubin kernicterus is a rare, but refractory cause of bilirubin-induced neurotoxicity in preterm neonates.[2] The term refers to bilirubin-induced neuronal damage at TB levels generally thought to be nonhazardous, that is, those below double volume exchange transfusion (DVET) thresholds. The CNS bilirubin exposure, however, is neurotoxic, suggesting either (i) an albumin problem, that is, an abnormally low serum albumin and/or impaired albumin-bilirubin binding that results in a hazardous UB concentration; and/or (ii) a vulnerable neuronal pool resulting from cellular immaturity coupled with antecedent or concurrent insults that potentiate bilirubin neurotoxicity.[2] Oftentimes both an albumin problem and a vulnerable neuronal pool are evident in a given neonate with low-bilirubin kernicterus, suggesting this is a 2-hit or multihit phenomenon.[2] **Table 1** shows the frequency of adverse conditions in recent case reports.[2,6,7,49–53]

As highlighted in **Table 1**, one of the more common clinical conditions associated with low-bilirubin kernicterus is hypoalbuminemia, often at concentrations well below the standard critical serum albumin neurotoxicity risk factor criterion of less than 2.5 g/dL for preterm neonates.[44,54,55] Indeed, trough serum albumin levels in the low-bilirubin kernicterus case series of Govaert and colleagues[6] ranged from 1.3 to 1.9 g/dL. A modestly elevated TB, with this degree of hypoalbuminemia, holds the potential for neurotoxicity given the limited albumin-bilirubin binding capacity dictated by the very low serum albumin *alone*, independent of any adverse alteration in albumin-bilirubin binding affinity.

In this regard, it is notable that every neonate in the case series of Govaert and colleagues[6] of low-bilirubin kernicterus demonstrated elevated bilirubin/albumin ratios (BAR) that met or exceeded the DVET treatment thresholds set forth by Ahlfors[54] and used in the recent Bilirubin Albumin Ratio Trial (BARTrial)[56] (**Table 2**). In contrast, the TB treatment threshold for DVET was either not met or exceeded only after the BAR.

These findings suggest that although the BAR is an imperfect surrogate of free bilirubin and CNS bilirubin exposure, during extreme hypoalbuminemia the BAR may become a meaningful proxy of bilirubin neurotoxicity risk. Prior studies showing

Table 1
Adverse conditions in case reports of low-bilirubin kernicterus (2001–2013)

Reference	Serum Albumin <2.5 g/dL	BAR for DVET Exceeded	Infection/ Inflammation	Comorbid CNS Injury[a]	Preterm Gestation[d]	Two or More Risk Factors
Govaert et al,[6] 2003[b]	5/5	5/5	2/5	4/5	$25^{4/7}$–$29^{0/7}$	5/5
Odutolu & Emmerson,[49] 2013	1/1	1/1	1/1	0/1	$36^{6/7}$	1/1
Moll et al,[50] 2011	N/A	N/A	1/2	2/2	$24^{0/7}$–$26^{0/7}$	2/2
Okumura et al,[51] 2009[b]	N/A	N/A	N/A	1/5	$25^{0/7}$–$31^{0/7}$	1/5
Gkoltsiou et al,[7] 2008[c]	N/A	N/A	3/3	3/3	$27^{0/7}$–$35^{0/7}$	3/3
Sugama et al,[52] 2001	N/A	N/A	1/2	1/2	$31^{0/7}$–$34^{0/7}$	2/2
Kamei et al,[53] 2012	1/2	1/2	N/A	0/2	$24^{6/7}$–$27^{0/7}$	1/2
Adverse condition per cases	7/8	7/8	8/13	11/20	20/20	15/20

Numbers are likely an underestimate because conditions were not systematically screened across all the studies.

Abbreviations: IVH, intraventricular hemorrhage; N/A, not available; PVL, periventricular leukomalacia.
[a] PVL, IVH (grade II, III, and/or IV), hydrocephalus ex vacuo.
[b] Only 5 of 8 reported cases of kernicterus met the definition of low-bilirubin kernicterus.
[c] Only 3 infants in reported cases of kernicterus met the definition of low-bilirubin kernicterus.
[d] All infants were preterm (<$37^{0/7}$ wks GA), gestational age, or ranges as shown.
Adapted from Watchko JF, Maisels MJ. The enigma of low bilirubin kernicterus in premature infants: why does it still occur, and is it preventable? Semin Perinatol 2014;38:398; with permission.

Table 2
Bilirubin:albumin ratio trial phototherapy and exchange transfusion criteria

	Phototherapy				Exchange Transfusion			
	Standard Risk		High Risk		Standard Risk		High Risk	
Birth Weight (g)	TB	B/A	TB	B/A	TB	B/A	TB	B/A
<1000	5.8	2.3	5.8	2.3	9.9	3.9	9.9	3.9
1000–1250	8.7	3.5	5.8	2.3	12.8	5.1	9.9	3.9
1250–1500	11.1	3.7	8.7	2.9	15.2	6.1	12.8	5.1
1500–2000	12.8	4.2	11.1	3.7	16.9	6.8	15.2	6.1
2000–2500	14.0	4.6	12.8	4.2	18.1	7.2	16.9	6.8

At 48 h of postnatal age and older.
High risk: asphyxia, hypoxemia, acidosis, hemolysis, neurologic deterioration (sepsis, meningitis, intracranial hemorrhage > grade 2).
TB is expressed in milligrams per deciliter and bilirubin:albumin ratio (B/A) ratio is expressed as milligrams per gram.
From Hulzebos CV, Dijk PH, van Imhoff DE, et al. The bilirubin albumin ratio in the management of hyperbilirubinemia in preterm infants to improve neurodevelopmental outcome: a randomized controlled trial—the BARTrial. PLoS One 2014;9:e99466.

no difference in outcomes between infants managed using the BAR versus TB are constrained by their small number of subjects with marked hypoalbuminemia. Indeed, the BAR will not improve neurotoxicity risk prediction when the albumin level is normal[56] or when the TB concentration is exceedingly high.[57] Initiation of phototherapy at lower treatment thresholds when hypoalbuminemia is present as detailed using the BAR in the BARTrial (see **Table 2**)[56] or the TB level in a recently recommended preterm hyperbilirubinemia management guideline[44] holds promise to reduce the incidence of low-bilirubin kernicterus.[6]

Hypoalbuminemia

The underlying pathophysiologic mechanisms and clinical conditions associated with hypoalbuminemia in neonates are outlined in **Table 3**.[58,59] Those most frequently encountered mechanisms include albumin loss and altered albumin distribution.[58,59] The latter refers to leakage of albumin from the intravascular space into the extravascular, extracellular interstitial space reported in association with several conditions in sick preterm newborns (see **Table 3**). Significant albumin loss secondary to fetal perinatal hemorrhage is also an important contributor to marked hypoalbuminemia and is seen in (i) fetal maternal transfusion; (ii) the donor twin in twin-twin transfusion syndrome (TTTS)[60] and the twin anemia-polycythemia sequence (TAPS)[61]; and (iii) neonatal anemia associated with malformations of the placenta and cord.[62] For example, serum albumin levels of less than 2.5 g/dL were observed in half and less than 2.0 g/dL in almost one-quarter of donors in TTTS.[60] Whenever anemia is present in the immediate neonatal period, measurement of the albumin concentration is prudent.

Subtle kernicterus (bilirubin-induced neurologic dysfunction)

Although bilirubin-induced neurologic damage is most often thought of in terms of classic severe adverse neuromotor and auditory sequelae, it is postulated that bilirubin neurotoxicity may manifest as other less severe neurodevelopmental disabilities, a condition termed subtle kernicterus or BIND.[1,63–65] BIND is defined by a constellation of "subtle neurodevelopmental disabilities without the classical findings

Table 3
Mechanisms of hypoalbuminemia and associated clinical conditions in neonates

Mechanism	Clinical Conditions
1. Decreased synthesis	Hepatic failure, sepsis, inflammation
2. Increased catabolism	Critical illness
3. Abnormal loss	Hemorrhage • Fetal maternal hemorrhage • TTTS (donor) • TAPS (donor) • Surgical loss • Malformations of placenta and cord Nephrotic syndrome
4. Altered distribution between intravascular and extravascular space	Sepsis Necrotizing enterocolitis Inflammation Asphyxia Hydrops fetalis (nonimmune and immune) Isoimmune hemolytic disease of the newborn

Data from Uhing MR. The albumin controversy. Clin Perinatol 2004;31:475–88; and Nicholson JP, Wolmarans MR, Park GR. The role of albumin in critical illness. Br J Anaesth 2000;85:599–610.

of kernicterus that, after careful evaluation and exclusion of other possible etiologies, appear to be due to bilirubin neurotoxicity."[1] These purportedly include (i) mild to moderate disorders of movement (eg, incoordination, clumsiness, gait abnormalities, disturbances in static and dynamic balance, impaired fine motor skills, and ataxia); (ii) disturbances in muscle tone; and (iii) altered sensorimotor integration.[1,63–65] A putative association between postnatal hyperbilirubinemia and an increased risk of cognitive dysfunction (eg, lower intelligence quotient) and a range of neuropsychiatric syndromes including attention deficit-hyperactivity disorder, autism, and schizophrenia has also been alleged.[1,63–65] However, as with subtle kernicterus, the linkage between hyperbilirubinemia and their genesis remains uncertain and a source of continued study and debate.

The possible neuroanatomical basis for subtle kernicterus is unclear, but investigators have suggested a range of subcortical neuropathology, including the cerebellum and cerebellar projections.[66–68] The focus on the cerebellum derives from the following: (i) the cerebellum is vulnerable to bilirubin-induced injury, perhaps the most vulnerable region within the CNS; (ii) infants with cerebellar injury exhibit a neuromotor phenotype similar to BIND; and (iii) the cerebellum has extensive bidirectional circuitry projections to motor and nonmotor regions of the brainstem and cerebral cortex that impact a variety of neuromotor behaviors.[66,68]

Studies are needed to more precisely define the neural network abnormalities in infants with a BIND phenotype using advanced neuroimaging technology to shed light on its pathogenesis, including the putative role of bilirubin in the outcome.[5] Until these and other clinical investigations are completed, a causal linkage between bilirubin and subtle neurodevelopmental disabilities remains speculative.

REFERENCES

1. Shapiro SM. Kernicterus. In: Stevenson DK, Maisels MJ, Watchko JF, editors. Care of the jaundiced neonate. New York: McGraw Hill; 2012. p. 229–42.
2. Watchko JF, Maisels MJ. The enigma of low bilirubin kernicterus in premature infants: why does it still occur, and is it preventable? Semin Perinatol 2014;38: 397–406.
3. Ahdab-Barmada M. The neuropathology of kernicterus: definitions and debate. In: Maisels MJ, Watchko JF, editors. Neonatal jaundice. Amsterdam: Harwood Academic Publishers; 2000. p. 75–88.
4. Penn AA, Enzmann DR, Hahn JS, et al. Kernicterus in a full term infant. Pediatrics 1994;93:1003–6.
5. Wisnowski JL, Panigrahy A, Painter M, et al. Magnetic resonance imaging of bilirubin encephalopathy: current limitations and future promise. Semin Perinatol 2014;38:422–8.
6. Govaert P, Lequin M, Swarte R, et al. Changes in globus pallidus with (pre) term kernicterus. Pediatrics 2003;112:1256–63.
7. Gkoltsiou K, Tzoufi M, Counsell S, et al. Serial brain MRI and ultrasound findings: relation to gestational age, bilirubin level, neonatal neurologic status and neurodevelopmental outcome in infants at risk of kernicterus. Early Hum Dev 2008;84: 829–38.
8. Watchko JF, Tiribelli C. Bilirubin-induced neurologic damage—mechanisms and management approaches. N Engl J Med 2013;369:2012–30.
9. Brites D, Bhutani VK. Pathways involving bilirubin and other brain-injuring agents. In: Dan B, Mayston M, Paneth N, et al, editors. Cerebral palsy: science and clinical practice. London: Mac Keith Press; 2014. p. 131–49.

10. Brites D, Brito MA. Bilirubin toxicity. In: Stevenson DK, Maisels MJ, Watchko JF, editors. Care of the jaundiced neonate. New York: McGraw Hill; 2012. p. 115–1423.
11. Hansen TWR. The pathophysiology of bilirubin toxicity. In: Maisels MJ, Watchko JF, editors. Neonatal jaundice. Amsterdam: Harwood Academic Publishers; 2000. p. 89–104.
12. Watchko JF. Kernicterus and the molecular mechanisms of bilirubin-induced CNS injury in newborns. Neuromolecular Med 2006;8:513–29.
13. Hansen TWR, Bratlid D. Bilirubin and brain toxicity. Acta Paediatr Scand 1986;75: 513–22.
14. Zucker SD, Goessling W, Bootle EJ, et al. Localization of bilirubin in phospholipid bilayers by parallax analysis of fluorescence quenching. J Lipid Res 2001;42: 1377–88.
15. Wennberg RP, Ahlfors CE, Rasmussen LF. The pathochemistry of kernicterus. Early Hum Dev 1979;3:353–72.
16. Brito MA, Brites D, Butterfield DA. A link between hyperbilirubinemia, oxidative stress and injury to neocortical synaptosomes. Brain Res 2004;1026:33–43.
17. Rodrigues CM, Sola S, Castro RE, et al. Perturbation of membrane dynamics in nerve cells as an early event during bilirubin-induced apoptosis. J Lipid Res 2002;43:885–94.
18. Ly EM, Cameron G, Tang N, et al. Choline reduces bilirubin inhibition of L1 cell adhesion molecule (L1) mediated neurite outgrowth. EPAS 2015;2912:503.
19. Johnston MV. Excitotoxicity in perinatal brain injury. Brain Pathol 2005;15:234–40.
20. Slemmer JE, De Zeeuw CI, Weber JT. Don't get too excited: mechanisms of glutamate-mediated Purkinje cell death. Prog Brain Res 2005;148:367–90.
21. Johnston MV, Hoon AH. Possible mechanisms in infants for selective basal ganglia damage from asphyxia, kernicterus, or mitochondrial encephalopathies. J Child Neurol 2000;15:588–91.
22. Novelli A, Reilly JA, Lysko PG, et al. Glutamate becomes neurotoxic via NMDA receptors when intracellular energy levels are reduced. Brain Res 1988;451: 205–12.
23. Greenamyre T, Penney JB, Young AB, et al. Evidence for transient perinatal glutaminergic innervation of globus pallidus. J Neurosci 1987;7:1022–30.
24. McDonald JW, Shapiro SM, Silverstein FS, et al. Role of glutamate receptor-mediated excitotoxicity in bilirubin-induced brain injury in the Gunn rat model. Exp Neurol 1998;150:21–9.
25. Oakden WK, Moore AM, Blaser S, et al. 1H MR spectroscopic characteristic of kernicterus: a possible metabolic signature. AJNR Am J Neuroradiol 2005;26: 1571–4.
26. Brites D. The evolving landscape of neurotoxicity by unconjugated bilirubin: role of glial cells and inflammation. Front Pharmacol 2012;3:88.
27. Falcao AS, Fernandes A, Brito MA, et al. Bilirubin-induced inflammatory response, glutamate release, and cell death in rat cortical astrocytes is enhanced in younger cells. Neurolbiol Dis 2005;20:199–206.
28. Connolly AM, Volpe JJ. Clinical features of bilirubin encephalopathy. Clin Perinatol 1990;17:371–9.
29. Kitamura M. Control of NF-κB and inflammation by the unfolded protein response. Int Rev Immunol 2011;30:304–15.
30. Yueh MF, Chen S, Nguyen N, et al. Developmental onset of bilirubin-induced neurotoxicity involves Toll-like receptor 2-dependent signaling in humanized UDP-glucuronosyltransferase1 mice. J Biol Chem 2014;289:4699–709.

31. Falcao AS, Silva RFM, Vaz AR, et al. Cross-talk between neurons and astrocytes in response to bilirubin: early beneficial effects. Neurochem Res 2013;38:644–59.

32. Liaury K, Miyaoka T, Tsumori T, et al. Morphological features of microglial cells in the hippocampal dentate gyrus of Gunn rat: a possible schizophrenia animal model. J Neuroinflammation 2012;9:56.

33. Liaury K, Miyaoka T, Tsumori T, et al. Minocycline improves recognition memory and attenuates microglial activity in Gunn rat: a possible hyperbilirubinemia-induced animal model of schizophrenia. Prog Neuropsychopharmacol Biol Psychiatry 2014;50:184–90.

34. Mueller K. Inflammation's yin-yang. Introduction. Science 2013;339:155.

35. Daood MJ, Hoyson M, Watchko JF. Lipid peroxidation is not the primary mechanism of bilirubin-induced neurologic dysfunction in jaundiced Gunn rat pups. Pediatr Res 2012;72:455–9.

36. Conlee JW, Shapiro SM, Churn SB. Expression of the alpha and beta subunits of Ca2+/calmodulin kinase II in the cerebellum of jaundiced Gunn rats during development: a quantitative light microscopic analysis. Acta Neuropathol 2000; 99:393–401.

37. Shaia WT, Shapiro SM, Heller AJ, et al. Immunohistochemical localization of calcium-binding proteins in the brainstem vestibular nuclei of the jaundiced Gunn rat. Hear Res 2002;173:82–90.

38. Spencer RF, Shaia WT, Gleason AT, et al. Changes in calcium-binding protein expression in the auditory brainstem nuclei of the jaundiced Gunn rat. Hear Res 2002;171:129–41.

39. Robert MC, Furlan G, Rosso N, et al. Alterations in the cell cycle in the cerebellum of hyperbilirubinemic Gunn rat: a possible link with apoptosis? PLoS One 2013;8: e79073.

40. Daood MJ, Azzuqa A, Watchko JF. Bilirubin-induced cytostatsis, G0/G1 cell cycle arrest, and apoptosis as function of increasing concentration and duration of exposure in vitro. E-PAS 2014;4525.1.

41. Damico K, Daood M, Sanders T, et al. Sonic hedgehog (SHH) signaling axis is not perturbed during development of cerebellar hypoplasia in the neonatal hyperbilirubinemic Gunn rat model of kernicterus. E-PAS 2015;1578.573.

42. Falcao AS, Silva RF, Pancadas S, et al. Apoptosis and impairment of neurite network by short exposure of immature rat cortical neurons to unconjugated bilirubin increase with cell differentiation and are additionally enhanced by an inflammatory stimulus. J Neurosci Res 2007;865:1229–39.

43. Biran V, Verney C, Ferriero DM. Perinatal cerebellar injury in human and animal models. Neurol Res Int 2012;2012:858929.

44. Maisels MJ, Watchko JF, Bhutani VK, et al. An approach to the management of hyperbilirubinemia in the preterm infant less than 35 weeks of gestation. J Perinatol 2012;32:660–4.

45. American Academy of Pediatrics Subcommittee on Hyperbilirubinemia. Clinical practice guideline: management of hyperbilirubinemia in the newborn infant 35 or more weeks of gestation. Pediatrics 2004;114:297–316.

46. Amin S, Bhutani VK, Watchko JF. Apnea in acute bilirubin encephalopathy. Semin Perinatol 2014;38:407–11.

47. Crosse VM, Meyer TC, Gerrard JW. Kernicterus and prematurity. Arch Dis Child 1955;30:501–8.

48. Johnson L, Bhutani VK, Karp K, et al. Clinical report from the pilot USA Kernicerus Registry (1992 to 2004). J Perinatol 2009;29:S25–45.

49. Odutolu Y, Emmerson AJ. Low bilirubin kernicterus with sepsis and hypoalbumi-naemia. BMJ Case Rep 2013. http://dx.doi.org/10.1136/bcr-2012-008042.
50. Moll M, Goelz R, Naegele T, et al. Are recommended phototherapy thresholds safe enough for extremely low birth weight (ELBW) infants? A report on 2 ELBW infants with kernicterus despite only moderate hyperbilirubinemia. Neonatology 2011;99:90–4.
51. Okumura A, Kidokoro H, Shoji H, et al. Kernicterus in preterm infants. Pediatrics 2009;123:e1052.
52. Sugama S, Soeda A, Eto Y. Magnetic resonance imaging in three children with kernicterus. Pediatr Neurol 2001;25:328–31.
53. Kamei A, Sasaki M, Akasaka M, et al. Proton magnetic resonance spectroscopic images in preterm infants with bilirubin encephalopathy. J Pediatr 2012;160: 342–4.
54. Ahlfors CE. Criteria for exchange transfusion in jaundiced newborns. Pediatrics 1994;93:488–94.
55. Bryla DA. Randomized, controlled trial of phototherapy for neonatal hyperbilirubine-mia. Development, design, and sample composition. Pediatrics 1985;75(Suppl): 387–92.
56. Hulzebos CV, Dijk PH, van Imhoff DE, et al. The bilirubin albumin ratio in the man-agement of hyperbilirubinemia in preterm infants to improve neurodevelopmental outcome: a randomized controlled trial—the BARTrial. PLoS One 2014;9:e99466.
57. Iskander I, Gamaleldin R, El Houchi S, et al. Serum bilirubin and bilirubin/albumin ratio as predictors of bilirubin encephalopathy. Pediatrics 2014;134:e1330–9.
58. Uhing MR. The albumin controversy. Clin Perinatol 2004;31:475–88.
59. Nicholson JP, Wolmarans MR, Park GR. The role of albumin in critical illness. Br J Anaesth 2000;85:599–610.
60. Verbeek L, Middeldorp JM, Hulzebos CV, et al. Hypoalbuminemia in donors with twin-twin transfusion syndrome. Fetal Diagn Ther 2013;33:98–102.
61. Verbeek L, Slaghekke F, Hulzebos CV, et al. Hypoalbuminemia in donors with twin anemia-polycythemia sequence: a matched case-control study. Fetal Diagn Ther 2013;33:241–5.
62. Oski FA. Anemia in the neonatal period. In: Oski FA, Naiman JL, editors. Hematologic problems in the newborn. Philadelphia: WB Saunders; 1982. p. 56–86.
63. Johnson LH, Bhutani VK, Brown AK. System-based approach to management of neonatal jaundice and prevention of kernicterus. J Pediatr 2002;140:396–403.
64. Shapiro SM. Definition of the clinical spectrum of kernicterus and bilirubin-induced neurologic dysfunction (BIND). J Perinatol 2005;25:54–9.
65. Bhutani VK, Johnson-Hamerman LJ. The clinical syndrome of bilirubin-induced neurologic dysfunction. Semin Fetal Neonatal Med 2015;20:6–13.
66. Koziol LF, Budding DE, Chidekel D. Hyperbilirubinemia:subcortical mechanisms of cognitive and behavioral dysfunction. Pediatr Neurol 2013;48:3–13.
67. Lunsing RJ, Pardoen WF, Hadders-Algra M. Neurodevelopment after moderate hyperbilirubinemia at term. Pediatr Res 2013;73:655–60.
68. Watchko JF, Painter MJ, Panigraphy A. Are the neuromotor disabilities of bilirubin-induced neurologic dysfunction (BIND) disorders related to the cerebellum and its connections? Semin Fetal Neonatal Med 2015;20:47–51.

Bilirubin-Induced Audiologic Injury in Preterm Infants

Cristen Olds, MD, John S. Oghalai, MD*

KEYWORDS

- Bilirubin • Preterm • Kernicterus • Auditory neuropathy • Hyperbilirubinemia
- Auditory brainstem response • Cochlea • Cochlear nucleus

KEY POINTS

- In preterm infants, bilirubin-induced auditory impairment occurs at total serum/plasma bilirubin (TB) levels that have traditionally been considered safe.
- TB levels do predict auditory manifestations of hyperbilirubinemia in the preterm population. Although unbound or free bilirubin seems to correlates better with clinical presentation, it is not readily available for use as a screening tool in the clinical setting.
- Bilirubin-induced auditory impairment primarily affects brainstem nuclei and the auditory nerve, causing auditory neuropathy spectrum disorder. Auditory brainstem response measurement is the gold standard diagnostic test.
- Although standardized guidelines exist for screening and management of hyperbilirubinemia in infants born at 35 weeks gestational age or later, guidelines for infants born earlier are expert-mediated in the absence of best evidence.

INTRODUCTION

Although hyperbilirubinemia affects most term and late preterm infants in the immediate postnatal period, it is generally modest and of little clinical significance.[1] However, a subset of hyperbilirubinemic infants ultimately experience bilirubin-induced neurologic dysfunction (BIND), a spectrum of neurologic injury that includes classic kernicterus, acute bilirubin encephalopathy (ABE), and isolated neural pathway dysfunction.[2,3]

Funding Source: This work was funded by NIH R01 DC010075 and R56 DC010164 (to J.S. Oghalai), and an HHMI Research Training Fellowship grant and Stanford Medical Scholars Research Program grant (to C. Olds).
Financial Disclosure: Neither of the authors has financial relationship relevant to this article to disclose.
Conflict of Interest: None of the authors has conflicts of interest to disclose.
Department of Otolaryngology – Head and Neck Surgery, Stanford University, 801 Welch Road, CA 94305, USA
* Corresponding author.
E-mail address: joghalai@stanford.edu

The auditory system is particularly sensitive to the effects of bilirubin, ranging from subtle abnormalities in hearing and speech processing to complete deafness.[4–7] Auditory pathway damage may occur at total serum/plasma bilirubin (TB) levels that were previously thought to be harmless and may occur in the absence of other signs of classic kernicterus.[8] In addition, preterm infants may exhibit clinical evidence of kernicterus at normal or marginally elevated TB levels.[9,10] Damage to the auditory system has long-reaching consequences for affected children because language development is intricately tied to auditory function. Even mild-to-moderate hearing loss can significantly affect a child's quality of speech acquisition.[11]

Further complicating the picture is that the current American Academy of Pediatrics guideline for management of hyperbilirubinemia (including the use of phototherapy and exchange transfusion) are for infants at least 35 weeks gestational age (GA).[12–14] Similar evidence-based institutional guidelines are not available for infants less than 35 weeks GA.

This article explores the mechanisms and manifestations of bilirubin-induced damage of the auditory system in preterm infants.

MECHANISMS OF BILIRUBIN-INDUCED NEUROLOGIC DAMAGE

Animal studies have shown that unconjugated bilirubin passively diffuses across cell membranes and the blood-brain barrier, and that bilirubin not removed by organic anion efflux pumps accumulates within the cytoplasm and becomes toxic.[15,16] Exposure of neurons to bilirubin results in increased oxidative stress and decreased neuronal proliferation,[17,18] and presynaptic neurodegeneration at central glutaminergic synapses.[19] Furthermore, bilirubin administration results in smaller spiral ganglion cell bodies, with decreased cellular density and selective loss of large cranial nerve VIII myelinated fibers.[20,21] When exposed to bilirubin, neuronal supporting cells have been found to secrete inflammatory markers that contribute to increased blood-brain barrier permeability and bilirubin loading.[15,16]

The jaundiced Gunn rat is the classic animal model of bilirubin toxicity. It is homozygous for a premature stop codon within the gene for UDP-glucuronosyltransferase family 1 (UGT1A1).[22] The resultant gene product has reduced bilirubin-conjugating activity, leading to a state of hyperbilirubinemia. Studies using this rat model have led to the concept that impaired calcium homeostasis is an important mechanism of neuronal toxicity, with reduced expression of calcium-binding proteins in affected cells being a sensitive index of bilirubin-induced neuronal damage.[23] Similarly, application of bilirubin to cultured auditory neurons from brainstem cochlear nuclei results in hyperexcitability and excitotoxicity.[24]

There is some evidence suggesting that distinct developmental windows exist such that the age at bilirubin exposure is the main determinant of long-term neurologic sequelae because it determines what structures will be actively developing at the time of exposure.[25] Compared with term infants, preterm infants are more prone to neurologic insult in the immediate postnatal period because these insults are more likely to occur during the peak of neural circuit formation. In addition, the sensory pathways undergo myelination earlier and faster than motor pathways, which may partially explain why an auditory-predominant kernicterus subtype is more common in neonates less than 34 weeks GA, in contrast to the classic motor-predominant subtype that is observed in infants born closer to term.[26]

PRETERM INFANTS ARE PARTICULARLY VULNERABLE TO BILIRUBIN-INDUCED NEUROLOGIC DAMAGE

Hyperbilirubinemia is one of many risk factors for neonatal hearing loss, including noisy neonatal intensive care unit (NICU) environments, aminoglycoside exposure, central nervous system (CNS) infection, and hypoxia at birth.[27–29] Prematurity itself is associated with an increased risk neurodevelopmental disability, including sensory and cognitive impairments.[30–32] Preterm infants are at greatly increased all-cause risk of hearing loss when compared with their term counterparts.[33]

Preterm infants are more prone to BIND than their term counterparts for several reasons. They are more prone to unconjugated hyperbilirubinemia because they have increased bilirubin production and a relative deficiency of UGT1A1 expression compared with term infants.[34,35] In addition, they exhibit relatively increased enterohepatic circulation, preventing bilirubin from being eliminated in the stool.[36]

Factors common among preterm infants, such as metabolic derangement, hypoxic-ischemic events, and infection, may effectively increase the bilirubin burden in the CNS by increasing the permeability of the blood-brain barrier and independently cause neuronal injury that is further compounded by the oxidative stresses of bilirubin. This may partially explain why preterm infants are more susceptible to bilirubin-induced neurotoxicity than term infants and experience neurologic sequelae at lower TB levels.[37–39]

There is evidence that even late preterm infants should not be treated the same as their term counterparts. In a retrospective study with a cohort of 125 infants, near-term neonates (defined as 34 [0/7] to 36 [6/7] wk) that were treated the same as term infants were found to disproportionately develop kernicterus compared with their term counterparts and experience higher rates of severe posticteric sequelae (82.7% in late preterm infants compared with 70.8% in term infants, $P<.01$).[40]

BILIRUBIN-INDUCED NEUROLOGIC DAMAGE AND THE AUDITORY BRAINSTEM RESPONSE

Brainstem cochlear nuclei are the first structures affected by elevated TB levels, followed by the auditory nerve, with higher neural centers involved last.[21] The cochlea does not seem to be directly affected by hyperbilirubinemia.[20] However, cochlear damage can occur as a result of the damage to the auditory nerve or cochlear brainstem nuclei,[41] perhaps through loss of transcription factors that these cells provide that are necessary to maintain normal cochlear function.[42]

The auditory brainstem response (ABR) provides an electrophysiologic means of assessing the ascending auditory pathway and localizing the lesions. The electric field generated by the compound firing of neurons permits tracking of the auditory signal as it travels from the cochlea through each of the brainstem nuclei in sequence.[43–45] Consistent with disease affecting the brainstem rather than the cochlea, jaundiced Gunn rats have decreased amplitudes of ABR waves II and III (corresponding to waves III and V in the human ABR) and have increased interwave intervals.[46] They also exhibit decreased amplitude of the binaural interaction component of the ABR, indicating abnormal input to the superior olivary complex.[47] Similar ABR abnormalities in neonates have been described, including reduced amplitudes and increased latencies of ABR waves III and V. At higher TB levels, both humans and animal models also demonstrate loss of ABR wave I.[48,49] For example, a study of 37 term infants found that abnormal ABR findings correlated better with free or unbound bilirubin (UB) levels greater than 1.0 μg/dL than to TB levels greater than 20 mg/dL.[50,51]

Premature infants are prone to abnormal myelination of the auditory pathway secondary to developmental disruption or various metabolic insults. Neonatal I to V interpeak latency, an index of auditory nerve myelination at 35 weeks GA, was found to have significant correlation with language development at 3 years of age (as measured using the Preschool Language Scale) in a prospective study of 80 ex-preterm children.[52] Decreasing GA is significantly associated with an increased prevalence of neonatal hearing loss from 1.2% to 7.5% (ie, diagnostic ABR >35 decibel hearing loss) in a study of 18,564 neonates of GA 24 to 31 weeks (P<.002).[53]

AUDITORY NEUROPATHY SPECTRUM DISORDER

Auditory neuropathy spectrum disorder (ANSD) is commonly defined by abnormal auditory neural function (altered or missing ABR waveforms) in the presence of normal cochlear microphonics (the field potential emanating from the receptor potential of hair cells) and otoacoustic emissions (OAEs; sounds emanating from the ear due to nonlinear force production by the outer hair cells).[43,44,54–58] Children suffering from ANSD may have pure tone thresholds ranging from mild to profound hearing loss, and the actual threshold levels can vary during sequential tests on different days.[55,59,60] Speech perception is typically worse than would be predicted by pure tone thresholds.[55,59,61] Clinically, patients exhibit difficulties with sound localization or speech discrimination when visual cues are absent.[24]

ANSD is commonly associated with progressive hyperbilirubinemia. More than 50% of children suffering from ANSD have a history of hyperbilirubinemia and/or anoxia in the neonatal period.[62] Nickisch and colleagues[63] found that among 15 children with TB levels greater than 20 mg/dL in the neonatal period, 53% of them were diagnosed with ANSD by ABR testing at a mean age of 5.6 years. Conversely, none of 15 children in the control group with normal TB levels had ABR findings suggestive of ANSD at follow-up. Similarly, Saluja and colleagues[64] found that among a cohort of 13 neonates with hyperbilirubinemia requiring exchange transfusion, 46% had bilateral ABR abnormalities consistent with ANSD. However, although in this study there was no relationship between peak TB level and ANSD, a correlation was found in another study of greater than 600 subjects.[65] Similarly, Martínez-Cruz and colleagues[66] found that of 102 children who underwent exchange transfusion for hyperbilirubinemia, 15% presented with sensorineural hearing loss by a mean age of 5.5 plus or minus 3.9 years. They also had a higher unconjugated serum bilirubin level than their peers without hearing loss. Hearing loss at the time of documented hyperbilirubinemia (serum TB>10–20 mg/dL, depending on the study) was diagnosed by ABR or automated ABR (AABR) in 9.0% to 73.3% of children,[64,67–70] whereas the prevalence of hearing loss later in life (at 2 mo to 2 y of age) was only 2% to 6.7%.[70–72]

SPEECH AND LANGUAGE DISORDERS

Although ANSD is the best-characterized auditory manifestation of hyperbilirubinemia, disorders of speech and language have also been described. It is expected that children with ANSD will suffer from language difficulties given that auditory deprivation during the critical period for language acquisition results in central auditory processing and language abnormality.[73] Described sequelae include auditory aphasia and imperceptions, word deafness, decreased binaural fusion and auditory learning, and behavioral problems.[24,41,74] Language delay may manifest as subtle learning disabilities and auditory processing problems; however, no correlations between peak TB level or duration of elevated TB exposure in the neonatal period and language delays later in life have been found.[75] In situations in which hearing loss occurs as a result of hyperbilirubinemia, the ultimate damage to language skills may be lessened through early identification and management of hearing problems to improve auditory processing and language development.[76,77] Because of the known risk of hearing loss after hyperbilirubinemia, these children tend to be followed with serial audiometry very closely for several years, permitting early diagnosis and aggressive intervention for hearing loss.

THE UTILITY OF TOTAL SERUM/PLASMA BILIRUBIN LEVELS IN SCREENING FOR BILIRUBIN-INDUCED NEUROLOGIC DAMAGE

Even in term infants, there is much controversy about what levels of TB are problematic, with thresholds at which treatment is begun ranging between 10 to 23.4 mg/dL in various studies.[68,71,78–80] A commonly-used threshold in term infants is a TB greater than 20 mg/dL, with 35% of infants above this cutoff experiencing ABR abnormalities.[78] Nevertheless, in multiple cohorts, ABR abnormalities in preterm-to-term neonates (24–42 wk GA) showed no correlation with TB levels.[67,81] In addition to a lack of correlation between ABR findings and TB levels, at least one study has shown no significant correlation between peak TB levels in the neonatal period and childhood language delay in a cohort of preterm infants.[75]

There is a growing body of evidence that UB levels are a better indicator of neurologic dysfunction[82] and auditory system damage[38,39,51] than TB, especially in preterm infants. The UB level describes how much unconjugated bilirubin is not bound to albumin in circulation and depends on factors such as the serum albumin level and the affinity of albumin for bilirubin. Preterm infants are more likely to be hypoalbuminemic than their term counterparts, and bilirubin-binding capacity (BBC) is also decreased in neonates who are afflicted with sepsis, hypoxia, or other serious illness.[83,84] BBC was found to be directly proportional to GA in a series of 152 preterm (23–31 wk GA) and very low birthweight infants (<1300 g).[83]

Hypoalbuminemia and sepsis were correlated with the onset of bilirubin encephalopathy at lower TB levels than in neonates without these risk factors (25.4 vs >31.5 mg/dL) in a prospective series of 249 newborns.[85] In addition, several commonly used medications (eg, sulfonamides, cephalosporins, beta-lactam antibiotics) have been found to significantly displace bilirubin by preferentially binding to albumin, effectively increasing the UB concentration while maintaining a low TB level.[38] Although this is academically useful information, testing of UB levels is only routinely carried out in research settings and there are no existing clinical guidelines allowing the use of UB levels to guide management.

BENEFITS AND DRAWBACKS OF NEWBORN HEARING SCREENING

Hearing screening is an important aspect of diagnosing BIND-related auditory damage, with ABR being the test of choice.[68,80,86–88] An ABR test is performed by an audiologist and involves the presentation of tone stimuli at different frequencies. Electrodes are placed on the head to record the electric field evoked by the sound stimuli. The sound intensity is then varied to determine the minimum intensity required to evoke a neural response. This is called the threshold. By varying the frequency of the sound stimulus, auditory thresholds can be determined across the frequency spectrum.

Performing a diagnostic ABR is an involved process that can take an hour or more. To meet the demand to screen a large number of newborns, the AABR screening technique has been widely adopted in the United States. The AABR test works by presenting click stimuli at a moderately quiet level while the brainstem response is measured. The machine analyzes the response and gives either a pass (presence of ABR to the click) or refer (absence of ABR and need for a full follow-up diagnostic ABR test). Because the AABR is automated, it is quick and can be performed by a screener who does not need the comprehensive educational background and certification of a pediatric audiologist.

However, the AABR is not perfect and may miss infants with results that are not sufficiently abnormal to trigger a refer reading. Additionally, screening tests carried out soon after birth may occur before TB levels have increased to their peak levels and caused hearing loss.[89] This can lead to false-negative results; therefore, these children may not obtain follow-up that may allow diagnosis and treatment of subtle hearing and central auditory processing abnormalities. The prevalence of bilirubin neurotoxicity as a cause of audiological dysfunction may be underestimated if the TB alone is used to assess the severity of newborn hyperbilirubinemia, especially in the preterm population in which TB is particularly unhelpful for predicting neurologic outcomes.[81]

Despite the drawbacks of automated newborn hearing screening, it remains substantially better than OAE screening, which only tests for cochlear hearing loss. ANSD is usually completely missed by this test and it should not be used to screen children with hyperbilirubinemia.

IS BILIRUBIN-INDUCED NEUROLOGIC DAMAGE AUDITORY DAMAGE REVERSIBLE?

There is much interest in the potential for reversibility of BIND-related auditory dysfunction and there is growing evidence for reversibility of ABR abnormalities in animal models with the administration of albumin infusions.[38,39,90,91] Additionally, mild ABR abnormalities in infants may reverse with intervention by phototherapy and exchange transfusion, and some abnormalities resolve simply with the passage of time. In a prospective study of 56 infants with TB levels of at least 15 mg/dL (compared with 24 infants with normal TB levels), Nakamura and colleagues[50] found that prolonged latencies of ABR peaks I and V resolved after exchange transfusion. It has been suggested that diagnostic ABR is sensitive to the earliest manifestations of neurotoxicity, and that lowering TB at the time of abnormal ABR may allow only transient toxic neural effects[8]; however, there have been no controlled trials to confirm this.

Neonates with ANSD and a history of hyperbilirubinemia are often referred for cochlear implantation. In the authors' experience, this is the one scenario in which sensorineural hearing loss may spontaneously reverse. We have seen this occur only twice in over 1300 children evaluated for deafness, with approximately 90 of them having ANSD.[4,5] Both patients maintained normal OAEs and experienced full recovery of ABR waveforms before the age of 12 months. Thus, our typical clinical paradigm is to wait until this age before performing cochlear implantation in any child with ANSD. However, if a child with ANSD loses their OAEs during the first year of life, this indicates that secondary cochlear damage has occurred. In this unfortunate situation, the cochlear hearing loss will not reverse.

SUMMARY

BIND-related auditory damage includes a spectrum of manifestations on the auditory neuropathy spectrum with varying long-term severity, the full extent of which has yet to be fully characterized. Auditory system damage commonly occurs at plasma bilirubin concentrations that are below commonly-used therapeutic thresholds in preterm infants, possibly because the timing of sensory pathway myelination coincides with the immediate postnatal period in these infants. The damage to the auditory system caused by bilirubin in the preterm population is further exacerbated in the presence of concomitant infection, hypoxia, or other metabolic derangements. Guidelines for differential screening of premature infants are not well-defined, and the full impact of hyperbilirubinemia on the preterm population remains largely unknown. In addition to the paucity of literature focusing on preterm infants, most existing studies are observational, relatively small, and lack control groups. Although ABR is an imperfect screening tool in this population, there is some evidence that the technique (especially serial ABR screening) may be useful in identifying auditory BIND-related auditory damage in its earliest stages and preventing long-term neurodevelopmental deficits.

REFERENCES

1. Bhutani VK, Stark AR, Lazzeroni LC, et al. Predischarge screening for severe neonatal hyperbilirubinemia identifies infants who need phototherapy. J Pediatr 2013;162:477–82.e1.
2. Bhutani VK, Stevenson DK. The need for technologies to prevent bilirubin-induced neurologic dysfunction syndrome. Semin Perinatol 2011;35:97–100.
3. Olds C, Oghalai JS. Audiologic impairment associated with bilirubin-induced neurologic damage. Semin Fetal Neonatal Med 2015;20:42–6.
4. Lin JW, Chowdhury N, Mody A, et al. Comprehensive diagnostic battery for evaluating sensorineural hearing loss in children. Otol Neurotol 2011;32:259–64.
5. Jerry J, Oghalai JS. Towards an etiologic diagnosis: assessing the patient with hearing loss. Adv Otorhinolaryngol 2011;70:28–36.
6. Oghalai JS, Chen L, Brennan ML, et al. Neonatal hearing loss in the indigent. Laryngoscope 2002;112:281–6.
7. Cristobal R, Oghalai JS. Hearing loss in children with very low birth weight: current review of epidemiology and pathophysiology. Arch Dis Child Fetal Neonatal Ed 2008;93:F462–8.
8. Smith CM, Barnes GP, Jacobson CA, et al. Auditory brainstem response detects early bilirubin neurotoxicity at low indirect bilirubin values. J Perinatol 2004;24:730–2.
9. Morioka I, Nakamura H, Koda T, et al. Serum unbound bilirubin as a predictor for clinical kernicterus in extremely low birth weight infants at a late age in the neonatal intensive care unit. Brain Dev 2015;37:753–7.
10. Watchko JF, Maisels MJ. The enigma of low bilirubin kernicterus in premature infants: why does it still occur, and is it preventable? Semin Perinatol 2014;38:397–406.
11. Dlouha O, Novak A, Vokral J. Central auditory processing disorder (CAPD) in children with specific language impairment (SLI). Central auditory tests. Int J Pediatr Otorhinolaryngol 2007;71:903–7.
12. American Academy of Pediatrics Subcommittee on Hyperbilirubinemia. Management of hyperbilirubinemia in the newborn infant 35 or more weeks of gestation. Pediatrics 2004;114:297–316.
13. Maisels MJ, Bhutani VK, Bogen D, et al. Management of hyperbilirubinemia in the newborn infant 35 or more weeks of gestation: an update with clarifications. Pediatrics 2009;124:1193–8.
14. Bhutani VK, Committee on Fetus and Newborn. Phototherapy to prevent severe neonatal hyperbilirubinemia in the newborn infant 35 or more weeks of gestation. Pediatrics 2011;128:e1046–52.

15. Brites D, Fernandes A, Falcão AS, et al. Biological risks for neurological abnormalities associated with hyperbilirubinemia. J Perinatol 2009;29(Suppl 1):S8–13.
16. Brites D. The evolving landscape of neurotoxicity by unconjugated bilirubin: role of glial cells and inflammation. Front Pharmacol 2012;3:88.
17. Brito MA, Lima S, Fernandes A, et al. Bilirubin injury to neurons: contribution of oxidative stress and rescue by glycoursodeoxycholic acid. Neurotoxicology 2008;29:259–69.
18. Fernandes A, Falcão AS, Abranches E, et al. Bilirubin as a determinant for altered neurogenesis, neuritogenesis, and synaptogenesis. Dev Neurobiol 2009;69:568–82.
19. Haustein MD, Read DJ, Steinert JR, et al. Acute hyperbilirubinaemia induces presynaptic neurodegeneration at a central glutamatergic synapse. J Physiol 2010;588:4683–93.
20. Belal AJ. Effect of hyperbilirubinemia on the inner ear in Gunn rats. J Laryngol Otol 1975;89:259–65.
21. Uziel A, Marot M, Pujol R. The Gunn rat: an experimental model for central deafness. Acta Otolaryngol 1983;95:651–6.
22. Ikushiro S. Takashi Iyanagi. UGT1 gene complex: from Gunn rat to human. Drug Metab Rev 2010;42:14–22.
23. Spencer RF, Shaia WT, Gleason AT, et al. Changes in calcium-binding protein expression in the auditory brainstem nuclei of the jaundiced Gunn rat. Hear Res 2002;171:129–41.
24. Shapiro S, Nakamura H. Bilirubin and the auditory system. J Perinatol 2001;21(Suppl 1):S52–5.
25. Brites D, Fernandes A. Bilirubin-induced neural impairment: a special focus on myelination, age-related windows of susceptibility and associated co-morbidities. Semin Fetal Neonatal Med 2015;20:14–9.
26. Shapiro SM. Chronic bilirubin encephalopathy: diagnosis and outcome. Semin Fetal Neonatal Med 2010;15:157–63.
27. Coenraad S, Goedegebure A, van Goudoever JB, et al. Risk factors for sensorineural hearing loss in NICU infants compared to normal hearing NICU controls. Int J Pediatr Otorhinolaryngol 2010;74:999–1002.
28. Yoshikawa S, Ikeda K, Kudo T, et al. The effects of hypoxia, premature birth, infection, ototoxic drugs, circulatory system and congenital disease on neonatal hearing loss. Auris Nasus Larynx 2004;31:361–8.
29. Boo NY, Oakes M, Lye MS, et al. Risk factors associated with hearing loss in term neonates with hyperbilirubinaemia. J Trop Pediatr 1994;40:194–7.
30. Johnson S, Evans TA, Draper ES, et al. Neurodevelopmental outcomes following late and moderate prematurity: a population-based cohort study. Arch Dis Child Fetal Neonatal Ed 2015;100:F301–8.
31. Brosco JP, Sanders LM, Dowling M, et al. Impact of specific medical interventions in early childhood on increasing the prevalence of later intellectual disability. JAMA Pediatr 2013;167:544–8.
32. Graziani LJ, Mitchell DG, Kornhauser M, et al. Neurodevelopment of preterm infants: neonatal neurosonographic and bilirubin studies. Pediatrics 1992;89:229–32.
33. Soleimani F, Zaheri F, Abdi F. Long-term neurodevelopmental outcome s after preterm birth. Iran Red Crescent Med J 2014;16:e17965.
34. Watchko JF, Maisels MJ. Jaundice in low birthweight infants: pathobiology and outcome. Arch Dis Child Fetal Neonatal Ed 2003;88:455–9.

35. Ullrich D, Feveryg J, Siegt A, et al. The influence of gestational age on bilirubin conjugation in newborns. Eur J Clin Invest 1991;21:83–9.

36. Poland RL, Odell GB. Physiologic jaundice: the enterohepatic circulation of bilirubin. N Engl J Med 1971;284:1–6.

37. Watchko J, Oski F. Kernicterus in preterm newborns: past, present, and future. Pediatrics 1992;90:707–15.

38. Amin SB. Clinical assessment of bilirubin-induced neurotoxicity in premature infants. Semin Perinatol 2004;28:340–7.

39. Amin SB, Ahlfors C, Orlando MS, et al. Bilirubin and serial auditory brainstem responses in premature infants. Pediatrics 2001;107:664–70.

40. Bhutani VK, Johnson L. Kernicterus in late preterm infants cared for as term healthy infants. Semin Perinatol 2006;30:89–97.

41. Matkin N, Carhart R. Auditory profiles associated with Rh incompatibility. Arch Otolaryngol 1966;84:502–13.

42. Maricich SM, Xia A, Mathes EL, et al. Atoh1-lineal neurons are required for hearing and for the survival of neurons in the spiral ganglion and brainstem accessory auditory nuclei. J Neurosci 2009;29:11123–33.

43. Xia A, Gao SS, Yuan T, et al. Deficient forward transduction and enhanced reverse transduction in the alpha tectorin C1509G human hearing loss mutation. Dis Model Mech 2010;3:209–23.

44. Oghalai JS. The cochlear amplifier: augmentation of the traveling wave within the inner ear. Curr Opin Otolaryngol Head Neck Surg 2004;12:431–8.

45. Oghalai JS. Chlorpromazine inhibits cochlear function in guinea pigs. Hear Res 2004;198:59–68.

46. Diamond I, Schmid R. Experimental bilirubin encephalopathy. The mode of entry of bilirubin-14C into the central nervous system. J Clin Invest 1966;45:678–89.

47. Shapiro S. Binaural effects in brainstem auditory evoked potentials of jaundiced Gunn rats. Hear Res 1991;53:41–8.

48. Shapiro SM. Acute brainstem auditory evoked potential abnormalities in jaundiced Gunn rats given sulfonamide. Pediatr Res 1988;23:306–10.

49. Shapiro SM. Reversible brainstem auditory evoked potential abnormalities in jaundiced Gunn rats given sulfonamide. Pediatr Res 1993;34:629–33.

50. Nakamura H, Takada S, Shimabuku R. Auditory nerve and brainstem responses in newborn infants with hyperbilirubinemia. Pediatrics 1985;75:703–8.

51. Funato M, Tamai H, Shimada S, et al. Vigintiphobia, unbound bilirubin, and auditory brainstem responses. Pediatrics 1994;93:50–3.

52. Amin SB, Vogler-Elias D, Orlando M, et al. Auditory neural myelination is associated with early childhood language development in premature infants. Early Hum Dev 2014;90:673–8.

53. van Dommelen P, Verkerk PH, van Straaten HL. Hearing loss by week of gestation and birth weight in very preterm neonates. J Pediatr 2015;166:840–3.e1.

54. Shapiro SM, Bhutani VK, Johnson L. Hyperbilirubinemia and kernicterus. Clin Perinatol 2006;33:387–410.

55. Starr A, Picton TW, Sininger Y, et al. Auditory neuropathy. Eur Arch Otorhinolaryngol 1996;119:741–53.

56. Xia A, Song Y, Wang R, et al. Prestin regulation and function in residual outer hair cells after noise-induced hearing loss. PLoS One 2013;8:e82602.

57. Choi CH, Oghalai JS. Perilymph osmolality modulates cochlear function. Laryngoscope 2008;118:1621–9.

58. Xia A, Visosky AM, Cho JH, et al. Altered traveling wave propagation and reduced endocochlear potential associated with cochlear dysplasia in the BETA2/NeuroD1 null mouse. J Assoc Res Otolaryngol 2007;8:447–63.
59. Zdanski CJ, Buchman CA, Roush PA, et al. Assessment and rehabilitation of children with auditory neuropathy. Int Congr Ser 2004;1273:265–8.
60. Rance G, Beer DE, Cone-Wesson B, et al. Clinical findings for a group of infants and young children with auditory neuropathy. Ear Hear 1999;20:238–52.
61. Kraus N, Özdamar Ö, Stein L, et al. Absent auditory brain stem response: peripheral hearing loss or brain stem dysfunction? Laryngoscope 1984;94:400–6.
62. Rance G. Auditory neuropathy/dys-synchrony and its perceptual consequences. Trends Amplif 2005;9:1–43.
63. Nickisch A, Massinger C, Ertl-Wagner B, et al. Pedaudiologic findings after severe neonatal hyperbilirubinemia. Eur Arch Otorhinolaryngol 2009;266:207–12.
64. Saluja S, Agarwal A, Kler N, et al. Auditory neuropathy spectrum disorder in late preterm and term infants with severe jaundice. Int J Pediatr Otorhinolaryngol 2010;74:1292–7.
65. Hulzebos CV, van Dommelen P, Verkerk PH, et al. Evaluation of treatment thresholds for unconjugated hyperbilirubinemia in preterm infants: effects on serum bilirubin and on hearing loss? PLoS One 2013;8:e62858.
66. Martínez-Cruz CF, García Alonso-Themann P, Poblano A, et al. Hearing and neurological impairment in children with history of exchange transfusion for neonatal hyperbilirubinemia. Int J Pediatr 2014;2014:605828.
67. Ahlfors CE, Parker AE. Unbound bilirubin concentration is associated with abnormal automated auditory brainstem response for jaundiced newborns. Pediatrics 2008;121:976–8.
68. Jiang ZD, Brosi DM, Wilkinson AR. Changes in BAER wave amplitudes in relation to total serum bilirubin level in term neonates. Eur J Pediatr 2009;168:1243–50.
69. Guo X, Pu X, An T, et al. Characteristics of brainstem auditory evoked potential of neonates with mild or moderate hyperbilirubinemia. Neural Regen Res 2007;2: 660–4.
70. Sharma P, Chhangani N, Meena K. Brainstem evoked response audiometry (BAER) in neonates with hyperbilirubinemia. Indian J Pediatr 2006;73:413–6.
71. Wong V, Chen W, Wong K. Short- and long-term outcome of severe neonatal nonhemolytic hyperbilirubinemia. J Child Neurol 2006;21:309–15.
72. Chen W, Wong V, Wong K. Neurodevelopmental outcome of severe neonatal hemolytic hyperbilirubinemia. J Child Neurol 2006;21:474–9.
73. Kral A. Auditory critical periods: a review from system's perspective. Neuroscience 2013;247:117–33.
74. Johnson L, Bhutani V, Brown A. System-based approach to management of neonatal jaundice and prevention of kernicterus. J Pediatr 2002;140:396–403.
75. Amin SB, Prinzing D, Myers G. Hyperbilirubinemia and language delay in premature infants. Pediatrics 2009;123:327–31.
76. Moeller MP. Early intervention and language development in children who are deaf and hard of hearing. Pediatrics 2000;106:e43.
77. Olds C, Pollonini L, Abaya H, et al. Cortical activation patterns correlate with speech understanding after cochlear implantation. Ear Hear 2015. [Epub ahead of print].
78. Akinpelu O, Waissbluth S, Daniel S. Auditory risk of hyperbilirubinemia in term newborns: a systematic review. Int J Pediatr Otorhinolaryngol 2013;77:898–905.
79. Boo NY, Rohani AJ, Asma A. Detection of sensorineural hearing loss using automated auditory brainstem-evoked response and transient-evoked otoacoustic

emission in term neonates with severe hyperbilirubinaemia. Singapore Med J 2008;49:209–14.

80. Gupta A, Mann S. Is auditory brainstem response a neurotoxicity marker? Am J Otolaryngol 1998;19:232–6.
81. Ahlfors CE, Amin SB, Parker AE. Unbound bilirubin predicts abnormal automated auditory brainstem response in a diverse newborn population. J Perinatol 2009; 29:305–9.
82. Daood MJ, McDonagh AF, Watchko JF. Calculated free bilirubin levels and neuro-toxicity. J Perinatol 2009;29:S14–9.
83. Bender GJ, Cashore WJ, Oh W. Ontogeny of bilirubin-binding capacity and the effect of clinical status in premature infants born at less than 1300 grams. Pediatrics 2007;120:1067–73.
84. Reading RF, Ellisb R, Fleetwoodb A. Plasma albumin and total protein in preterm babies from birth to eight weeks. Early Hum Dev 1990;22:81–7.
85. Gamaleldin R, Iskander I, Seoud I, et al. Risk factors for neurotoxicity in newborns with severe neonatal hyperbilirubinemia. Pediatrics 2011;128:e925–31.
86. Sheykholeslami K, Kaga K. Otoacoustic emissions and auditory brainstem responses after neonatal hyperbilirubinemia. Int J Pediatr Otorhinolaryngol 2000;52:65–73.
87. Jiang ZD, Wilkinson AR. Impaired function of the auditory brainstem in term neonates with hyperbilirubinemia. Brain Dev 2014;36:212–8.
88. Jiang ZD, Liu T, Chen C. Brainstem auditory electrophysiology is supressed in term neonates with hyperbilirubinemia. Eur J Paediatr Neurol 2014;18:193–200.
89. Shapiro SM, Popelka GR. Auditory impairment in infants at risk for bilirubin-induced neurologic dysfunction. Semin Perinatol 2011;35:162–70.
90. Agrawal VK, Shukla R, Misra PK, et al. Brainstem auditory evoked response in newborns with hyperbilirubinemia. Indian Pediatr 1998;35:513–8.
91. Vinodh M, Ambikapathy P, Aravind MA, et al. Reversibility of brainstem evoked response audiometry abnormalities at 3 months in term newborns with hyperbilir-ubinemia. Indian Pediatr 2014;51:134–5.

The Preterm Infant

A High-Risk Situation for Neonatal Hyperbilirubinemia Due to Glucose-6-Phosphate Dehydrogenase Deficiency

Michael Kaplan, MB ChB[a,b,]*, Cathy Hammerman, MD[a,b],
Vinod K. Bhutani, MD[c]

KEYWORDS

- Glucose-6-phosphate dehydrogenase deficiency • Prematurity • Hyperbilirubinemia
- Kernicterus • Bilirubin encephalopathy • Hemolysis • Bilirubin conjugation

KEY POINTS

- Glucose-6-phosphate dehydrogenase (G6PD) deficiency can be associated with sudden and acute episodes of unpredictable, severe, or extreme hyperbilirubinemia.
- Immaturity of the bilirubin conjugating system in preterm infants may exacerbate hyperbilirubinemia by slowing the bilirubin excretory process.
- Both prematurity and G6PD deficiency are independent risk factors for neonatal hyperbilirubinemia, and together they can act synergistically with the potential for bilirubin encephalopathy and kernicterus.
- Preterm infants and infants with hemolytic conditions are thought to be at increased risk for bilirubin neurotoxicity compared with term infants or those without hemolysis.
- Early screening for G6PD deficiency and vigilant observation for jaundice, both in hospital and after discharge home, should facilitate referral to a medical center before the development of acute bilirubin encephalopathy.

Disclosure: The authors of the article have no conflict of interest to disclose related to any of the material herein included.
[a] Faculty of Medicine, The Hebrew University of Jerusalem, Ein Kerem, P.O. Box 12271, Jerusalem, 9112102 Israel; [b] Department of Neonatology, Shaare Zedek Medical Center, PO Box 3235, Jerusalem 91031, Israel; [c] Department of Pediatrics, Stanford University School of Medicine, 750 Welch Road, Suite 315, Palo Alto, CA 94305, USA
* Corresponding author. Faculty of Medicine, The Hebrew University of Jerusalem, Ein Kerem, P.O. Box 12271, Jerusalem, 9112102 Israel.
E-mail address: mkaplan@mail.huji.ac.il

Clin Perinatol 43 (2016) 325–340
http://dx.doi.org/10.1016/j.clp.2016.01.008
0095-5108/16/$ – see front matter © 2016 Elsevier Inc. All rights reserved.

Box 1

Some population subgroups in North America with a high frequency of glucose-6-phosphate dehydrogenase deficiency relative to the background frequency

African American

Sephardic Jews (Middle Eastern origin)

Mediterranean Basin (Italy, Greece, Turkey, Syria)

Middle Eastern origin

India

China

INTRODUCTION

Glucose-6-Phosphate Dehydrogenase Deficiency and Prematurity as Coexisting Risk Factors for Neonatal Hyperbilirubinemia

Glucose-6-phosphate dehydrogenase deficiency: the scope of the problem

Glucose-6-phosphate dehydrogenase (G6PD) deficiency is the most frequent enzyme deficiency encountered in humans and is estimated to affect more than 300 million individuals worldwide.[1,2] No longer limited to its indigenous distribution, which included the Mediterranean Basin, Central and West Africa, the Middle East, and Asia, slave trade, migration patterns in the past and present, and current-day ease of travel have transformed G6PD deficiency into a potentially dangerous condition that can be encountered in virtually any corner of the globe. Not surprisingly, G6PD deficiency is an important contributor to severe hyperbilirubinemia and kernicterus in low- and middle-income, developing countries with a high frequency of the condition.[3] Even more disturbing is the fact that G6PD deficiency features prominently in series of newborns with bilirubin neurotoxicity reported from Western countries, which have developed and functional health care systems, including the United States, Canada, the United Kingdom, and Ireland.[4–6] Complacency on the part of health care workers that, because they live in a geographic area with a low indigenous frequency of G6PD deficiency and the condition is of no concern to them, is no longer valid. Although North America is regarded as a low G6PD-deficiency region (0.5% to 2.9% male incidence in the United States and <0.5% in Canada),[7] there are subgroups of the population with a high frequency and whose members are at increased risk for the potential complications of the condition. At the top of this list are African Americans, in whom the male frequency of G6PD deficiency is 11% to 13% (**Box 1**).[8]

Medical complications associated with glucose-6-phosphate dehydrogenase deficiency

Favism and acute hemolytic episodes Most G6PD-deficient individuals will lead completely normal lives and, unless tested for, be unaware that they have the condition (**Box 2**). Some foods, chemical substances, and drugs may contain oxidizing

---

Box 2

Main potentially dangerous medical conditions associated with glucose-6-phosphate dehydrogenase deficiency

- Favism
- Extreme neonatal hyperbilirubinemia with potential for bilirubin neurotoxicity
- Moderate neonatal hyperbilirubinemia

components or metabolites which may cause an oxidative reaction with severe hemolysis leading to acute anemia. Infections have been emphasized as a leading trigger of hemolysis.[1] The classic food trigger is the fava bean. Hemolysis and hyperbilirubinemia have been reported in nursing newborns whose mothers ate fava.[9] Some additional commonly encountered substances include the following:

- Antimalarial drugs
- Sulpha-containing antibacterials
- Naphthalene used for storing clothes
- Vitamin K3 preparations (vitamin K1 in common use today is safe)
- Menthol-containing umbilical potions
- Triple dye for umbilical antisepsis
- Henna application to the newborn or maternal skin

Avoidance of these agents by individuals known to be G6PD-deficient and by breast-feeding mothers of infants known to be G6PD-deficient will protect them from the scourges of the condition and allow them to live normal lives.[1]

Extreme neonatal hyperbilirubinemia The most potentially devastating condition associated with G6PD deficiency is that of extreme neonatal hyperbilirubinemia.[10] The hyperbilirubinemia may be of sudden onset and total serum/plasma bilirubin (TB) levels may increase with rapidity to dangerous levels. In some cases, a trigger of hemolysis may be identified (see above). In many cases, however, an offending agent cannot be isolated, but as the clinical picture is similar to those with recognized hemolytic triggers, it is presumed that the hemolysis is due to a trigger, albeit with a hidden identity. Frequently, changes in hematologic indices, commonly associated with hemolysis in older children and adults, are absent in G6PD-deficient newborns with rapidly rising TB concentrations, giving rise to the incorrect presumption that the hyperbilirubinemia is not hemolytic in origin. The hemolytic basis, however, was demonstrated in a premature (35 weeks gestation) newborn who returned to hospital with sudden onset of severe hyperbilirubinemia. Despite the absence of decreasing hematocrit or increasing reticulocyte values compared with the birth hospitalization, blood carboxyhemoglobin (COHb) (indicative of the rate of heme catabolism) was several-fold the normal range of term newborns.[11]

Moderate neonatal hyperbilirubinemia G6PD-deficient neonates frequently develop a more moderate form of hyperbilirubinemia, in the main responsive to phototherapy, but sometimes requiring exchange transfusion. The pathophysiology of this hyperbilirubinemia includes a combination of increased hemolysis[12] and a predilection for diminished bilirubin conjugation,[13] the result, at least in part, of an interaction with a $(TA)_7$ promoter polymorphism of the uridine diphosphate (UDP)-glucuronosyltransferase 1A1 gene (*UGT1A1*28*) associated with Gilbert syndrome.[14]

Prematurity: added risk for neonatal hyperbilirubinemia

Premature infants are at higher risk for neonatal hyperbilirubinemia and its consequent neurotoxic complications than that for term infants. The primary reason for this increased propensity is immaturity of the bilirubin-conjugating enzyme, UDP-glucuronosyltransferase 1A1 (UGT1A1), in the preterm infant. Low UGT1A1 activity is universal in term infants, in whom its activity is 1% of that of adults.[15] With diminishing gestational age (GA), the enzyme activity becomes progressively less active, with resultant increase in risk for developing hyperbilirubinemia and bilirubin neurotoxicity, even in late preterm (34^0 to 36^6 weeks GA) and early term (38 weeks GA) newborns. Increased bilirubin production due to hemolysis, along with limited compensatory mechanisms due to immaturity, places these infants at increased risk for bilirubin-associated mortality and morbidity. It is also thought that bilirubin has a greater tendency to cross the blood-brain barrier and enter vulnerable brain cells in preterm infants compared with their term counterparts. Indeed, "low-bilirubin" kernicterus may be encountered in preterm newborns whose TB levels remained below recommended values for institution of therapy.[16]

Data from the Pilot Kernicterus Registry attest to the increased risk of late prematurity for bilirubin neurotoxicity.[4] Although infants less than 35 weeks GA were excluded from analysis, case details reported in the Kernicterus Registry testify to the increased risk of bilirubin-associated mortality and morbidity in late preterm newborns. Overall, of the 125 newborns reported, 30 (24%) were 35 and 36 weeks GA. Of the 5 babies who died within the first postnatal week, 4 were less than 37 weeks GA. Fifty percent of those 35 and 36 weeks GA displayed apnea as a sign of acute bilirubin encephalopathy (ABE) compared with 33.8% of those 37 weeks or greater GA. This finding may be particularly vexing because apnea in a preterm infant can easily be misinterpreted and attributed merely to prematurity, thereby potentially delaying the diagnosis of bilirubin neurotoxicity.

Glucose-6-phosphate dehydrogenase deficiency and prematurity: a synergistic, potentially dangerous, combination

Both increased hemolysis and prematurity are factors increasing the risk of bilirubin neurotoxicity, that is, bilirubin encephalopathy may occur at lower levels of TB than in nonhemolyzing or term infants.[17,18] It stands to reason that in G6PD-deficient neonates, in the face of acute hemolysis with overproduction of bilirubin, immaturity of the bilirubin conjugating enzyme, UDP-glucuronosyltransferase 1A1 (UGT1A1), will act as a bottleneck to bilirubin elimination and predispose the infant to exceptionally high TB values. Statistics from an African American neonatal cohort illustrate the cumulative and synergistic effect of risk factors, including prematurity, breast-feeding, and G6PD deficiency, on the incidence of hyperbilirubinemia.[19] Overall, the incidence of any TB ≥95th percentile on the Bhutani hour-specific nomogram was 43/500 (8.6%). Prematurity (defined in this study as 35–37 weeks GA) in and of itself did not increase the risk significantly (8.8%, odds ratio [OR] 1.03, 95% confidence interval [CI] 0.46 to 2.30). In premature infants who were exclusively breastfed, the rate of hyperbilirubinemia increased to 12.8%, whereas infants of the same subgroup who were also G6PD-deficient had a 10-fold increase (60%) in the incidence of hyperbilirubinemia (OR 10.2, 95% CI 1.35–76.9).

Glucose-6-phosphate dehydrogenase deficiency, prematurity, and uridine diphosphate-glucuronosyltransferase 1A1 (TA)$_7$ gene promoter polymorphism: an even higher risk combination

Further increasing the potential danger may be an additional icterogenic factor, that of the UGT1A1 (TA)$_7$ gene promoter polymorphism (UGT1A1*28), associated with Gilbert syndrome and known to interact with G6PD deficiency to increase the incidence of hyperbilirubinemia in term and late preterm infants.[14] Synergistic heterozygosity for this gene combination was recently reported in a preterm (35 weeks GA) female newborn, heterozygotic for both the G6PD Mediterranean mutation and the UGT1A1*28, leading to extreme hyperbilirubinemia with fatal outcome.[20] African-descent individuals in the Americas[21] and Nigerian newborns[22] have been demonstrated to have a higher frequency of UGT1A1*28 than Caucasian counterparts. Premature infants of these groups with an inherent high frequency of G6PD deficiency may therefore be at especially high risk for bilirubin neurotoxicity in the event of an acute hemolytic crisis.

IMBALANCE BETWEEN BILIRUBIN PRODUCTION AND ELIMINATION: THE BASIS OF NEONATAL HYPERBILIRUBINEMIA
Imbalance Between Bilirubin Production and Conjugation Demonstrated Mathematically

The 2 major processes contributing to neonatal hyperbilirubinemia include bilirubin production and its elimination, the latter process including uptake into the hepatocyte, conjugation, and its excretion into the bowel via the bile. (In newborns, a third process is in effect, that of the enterohepatic circulation, further increasing the bilirubin pool and overloading the elimination systems.) Equilibrium between the bilirubin formation and elimination processes will ensure that the TB does not reach dangerous levels. Lack of equilibrium, with bilirubin production outweighing its elimination, is the pathophysiologic basis for hyperbilirubinemia. The relationship between bilirubin production and conjugation with the TB has been demonstrated mathematically (**Box 3**). The equation comprised an index composed of blood COHb, corrected for ambient carbon monoxide (COHbc), an accurate index of heme catabolism and therefore bilirubin production, divided by total conjugated bilirubin (TCB), expressed as a percentage of TB (TCB[%TB]), an index of bilirubin conjugation.[23] This equation allows the assessment of the combined role of bilirubin production and conjugation in their contribution to the TB. Low heme catabolism rate (bilirubin production) along with efficient bilirubin conjugation should result in a low index, whereas high production relative to conjugation should result in a higher index.

Production-conjugation index in glucose-6-phosphate dehydrogenase-normal newborns

In a cohort of Israeli newborns, COHbc values correlated directly with TB concentrations ($r = 0.38$), and TCB[%TB] correlated inversely with TB ($r = 0.40$). The production-conjugation index correlated positively with TB values ($r = 0.61$), the correlation value for the index being higher than that of either COHbc or TCB[%TB] individually.[23] The production-conjugation index confirmed that imbalance between production and conjugation of bilirubin plays an important role in the mechanism of neonatal bilirubinemia.

The production-conjugation index in glucose-6-phosphate dehydrogenase-deficient neonates

In the G6PD-deficient wing of the study, this index was again used to explore the contributions of bilirubin production and conjugation to the pathophysiology of hyperbilirubinemia in these neonates.[24] Fifty-one G6PD-deficient neonates were sampled at 51 ± 8 hours for COHbc and TCB[%TB], concurrently. The production-conjugation index and TB correlated positively ($r = 0.45$, $P = .002$). On further analysis, it was evident that COHbc values, while higher than those of the G6PD-normal cohort, did not correlate with TB ($r = 0.22$, $P = .15$), a phenomenon that had been previously demonstrated

---

Box 3
The "production-conjugation index"

Production–Conjugation Index: COHbc/TCB(%TB)
COHbc: Blood carboxyhemoglobin, corrected for ambient carbon monoxideTCB[%TB]: Total serum/plasma conjugated bilirubin (TCB) expressed as a percentage of total serum/plasma bilirubin (TB)

From Kaplan M, Muraca M, Vreman HJ, et al. Neonatal bilirubin production-conjugation imbalance: effect of glucose-6-phosphate dehydrogenase deficiency and borderline prematurity. Arch Dis Child Fetal Neonatal Ed 2005;90:F123; with permission.

in G6PD-deficient neonates.[12,25] On the other hand, TCB[%TB] did correlate inversely with TB ($r = -0.42$, $P = .004$), implying that increasing TB is modulated by diminishing conjugative activity (**Figs. 1** and **2**).

The greater risk of glucose-6-phosphate dehydrogenase-deficient premature newborns demonstrated mathematically

In the above-mentioned study, subanalysis of the newborns born prematurely (35–37 weeks GA) demonstrated the greater nature of risk of G6PD-deficient premature infants compared with their term counterparts.[24] On the one hand, TB concentrations at the time of sampling were only modestly increased in the premature infants, and there was a weak correlation between diminishing GA and TB. In contrast, the production-conjugation index was greater than 2-fold in the premature compared with term neonates (2.31 [2.12–3.08] versus 1.05 [0.53–1.81], median [interquartile range], $P = .003$). This difference was attributable to immaturity of the conjugation process: although COHbc values were similar between the preterm and term newborns, the conjugated bilirubin fraction TCB[%TB] was lower in the preterm group (0.39 [0.31–0.42] versus 0.74 [0.44–1.69] $P = .009$ [median, interquartile range]), implying immaturity of the conjugation process as the primary factor increasing the index in these infants.

The higher production-conjugation index values in the premature subset implied greater lack of equilibrium between these processes in that group. The stage is therefore set for placing these infants at especially high risk. It stands to reason that should the equilibrium be further compromised, either by an additional hemolytic event or by further conjugative compromise such as presence of *UGT1A1*28* (TA)$_7$ promoter polymorphism, or more extreme prematurity, the potential for extreme hyperbilirubinemia would be greater in the preterm G6PD-deficient newborn than in the term counterpart.

CLINICAL REPORTS OF HYPERBILIRUBINEMIA IN GLUCOSE-6-PHOSPHATE DEHYDROGENASE-DEFICIENT PRETERM NEWBORNS
Clinical Series

There is a dearth of systematic studies encompassing the role of G6PD deficiency in the pathophysiology of neonatal hyperbilirubinemia specifically in preterm infants. The high-risk nature of preterm, G6PD-deficient newborns for significant hyperbilirubinemia was apparent already in the pre-phototherapy era. Eshaghpour and colleagues[26] identified 10 of 87 (11.5%) African American infants admitted to a premature infant nursery in Philadelphia, PA to be G6PD-deficient. Six (60%) of these developed TB levels greater

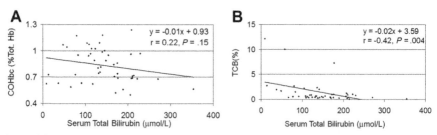

Fig. 1. (A) Regression analysis between blood COHb, corrected for inspired (room air) carbon monoxide (COHbc) and TB. (B) Regression analysis between TCB and TB. Hb, hemoglobin. (*From* Kaplan M, Muraca M, Vreman HJ, et al. Neonatal bilirubin production-conjugation imbalance: effect of glucose-6-phosphate dehydrogenase deficiency and borderline prematurity. Arch Dis Child Fetal Neonatal Ed 2005;90:F124; with permission.)

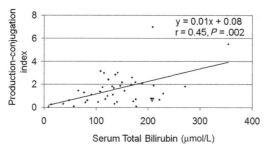

Fig. 2. Regression analysis between production-conjugation index and TB. (*From* Kaplan M, Muraca M, Vreman HJ, et al. Neonatal bilirubin production-conjugation imbalance: effect of glucose-6-phosphate dehydrogenase deficiency and borderline prematurity. Arch Dis Child Fetal Neonatal Ed 2005;90:F123–7; with permission.)

than 20 mg/dL, and exchange transfusion was performed in 5 (50%). In contrast, only 8 of the remaining 77 (10%) preterm infants underwent exchange transfusion.

Of 292 preterm Nigerian infants, 74 developed a TB ≥10 mg/dL of whom 13 (17.6%) were also G6PD-deficient.[27] Ashkenazi and colleagues[28] compared 17 preterm and low birthweight (BW) Israeli G6PD-deficient neonates with the next matched infant born with normal G6PD activity. Peak TB levels were significantly higher in the G6PD-deficient group than in controls (11.7 ± 1.4 versus 9.5 ± 2.1 mg/dL, P<.001). Use of phototherapy was somewhat, but not significantly, greater in the study group, whereas no infant in either group required exchange transfusion.

Case Reports

Some published case reports of hyperbilirubinemia in G6PD-deficient preterm infants have been alluded to in preceding paragraphs. Others will be summarized briefly in later discussion.

Costa and colleagues[29] describe a 32-week GA, 1350-g male second triplet who was hemizygous for G6PD Mediterranean. TB increased to 25 mg/dL at 78 hours despite phototherapy, and clinical evidence of ABE was apparent, necessitating exchange transfusion. No trigger of hemolysis could be identified. Hematologic indices did not indicate hemolysis (although these are poor indicators of increased heme catabolism in G6PD-deficient newborns).[11,30] Genetic studies excluded the presence of Gilbert syndrome. The investigators emphasized the role of immaturity of the bilirubin conjugating system in the pathogenesis of the hyperbilirubinemia and warn of the need to closely monitor TB levels in G6PD-deficient premature infants.

Several case reports emanating from Canada illustrate the effect of immigration on changing what was previously regarded as a country at low risk for G6PD deficiency (<0.5%) to one where G6PD deficiency may catch the pediatrician unaware. Nair and colleagues[31] described a 1320-g, 28-week GA premature infant who developed hyperbilirubinemia of hemolytic origin secondary to *Staphylococcus aureus* sepsis. The infant was G6PD-deficient. Bilateral cataracts, described in association with oxidative stress related to G6PD deficiency, developed in both eyes and required surgery. The investigators caution that cataracts should be monitored for in premature, G6PD-deficient infants with hemolytic episodes.

Lodha and colleagues[32] describe twins, one male and one female, born at 33 weeks GA who developed sudden onset of severe hyperbilirubinemia following episodes of enteritis due to *Clostridium difficile*. G6PD activity in both infants was low. The investigators suggest that the clostridium infection was responsible for inducing hemolysis with the resultant severe hyperbilirubinemia.

Turbendian and Perlman[33] in New York describe anemia, moderate hyperbilirubinemia, and prolonged jaundice in 31-week GA triplets born to a mother of African-Caribbean descent. G6PD activity by qualitative methodology was undetectable.

Shah and Yeo[34] report sudden onset of hyperbilirubinemia that progressed despite phototherapy and was, therefore, suggestive of hemolysis, requiring exchange transfusion, in an 1800-g, 34 week GA, male infant, first triplet born to Chinese parents in Singapore. No trigger of hemolysis was identified. Surprisingly, despite being exposed to the identical environmental factors, the second triplet, also a male infant and G6PD-deficient, and the third, a female infant with a G6PD level in the carrier range, developed only moderate hyperbilirubinemia responsive to phototherapy. These investigators emphasize that this G6PD-deficient preterm infant may have been at especial high risk for hemolysis and hyperbilirubinemia as a result of shortened red blood cell (RBC) lifespan, rendering these cells susceptible to oxidative damage, even in the absence of an identified trigger of hemolysis. They also emphasize that the hyperbilirubinemia may have been exacerbated by further combination with breast-feeding, immaturity of the bilirubin conjugation system, and possible interaction with UGT1A1*28[14] (although not actually studied for in this patient).

Tanphaichitr and colleagues[35] studied the incidence of hyperbilirubinemia 505 male newborns in Bangkok, Thailand, of whom 12% were G6PD-deficient. Hyperbilirubinemia requiring phototherapy was more prevalent in the G6PD-deficient newborns than in controls. It is noteworthy that the only infant in this series that required exchange transfusion was a premature G6PD-deficient newborn who had severe sepsis and succumbed.

Because it is an X-linked condition, female infants may be either homozygous for G6PD deficiency, homozygous G6PD-normal, or heterozygous.[1,10] In the past, heterozygotes were regarded as having sufficient G6PD activity to protect them from the dangers of G6PD activity.[7] However, hemolysis and hyperbilirubinemia have been reported in term G6PD heterozygotes,[36] while there have recently been reports of severe hyperbilirubinemia in preterm infants heterozygous for the G6PD Mediterranean mutation.[37] Kaplan and colleagues[36] described 2 female preterm infants: one (34 weeks GA), which developed sudden onset of hyperbilirubinemia requiring exchange transfusion while still hospitalized in the premature unit; the second (35 weeks GA), which was readmitted with a TB of 30 mg/dL and underwent exchange transfusion. Hemolysis was confirmed in the readmitted infant by demonstrating pre-exchange blood COHbc of 1.69%, more than twice the normal value of 0.69 ± 0.19% for heterozygote newborns sampled from the same nursery. A fatal case report of a heterozygote has already been cited above.[20]

The reason for hemolysis occurring in heterozygotes is that a large number of RBCs in any heterozygote will be G6PD-deficient. Biochemical enzyme assays measure a sample containing both G6PD-deficient and normal RBCs, and the average result is usually in the intermediate range. However, the affected RBCs in a heterozygotic individual harbor a not insignificant amount of potential bilirubin. Hemolysis of these cells may release sufficient quantities of heme to be catabolized to bilirubin. Immaturity of UGT1A1 in preterm infants (possibly exacerbated by UGT1A1*28) may be additive to the effect of hemolysis in potentiating severe hyperbilirubinemia.

DIAGNOSIS OF GLUCOSE-6-PHOSPHATE DEHYDROGENASE DEFICIENCY IN PREMATURE INFANTS
Glucose-6-Phosphate Dehydrogenase-Adequate Premature Infants

In general, it would appear that, in the normal range, term infants have higher G6PD activity than the normal range of 7 to 10 U/g Hb in adults.[38] This range has been demonstrated both in Israeli newborns, presumably with the G6PD Mediterranean mutation, and in African Americans, presumably to be G6PD A⁻.[39-41] The reason is most likely the high number of young RBCs with elevated G6PD activity in the newborn.

Few comprehensive studies of G6PD enzyme activity in preterm infants have been performed. Early studies were inconsistent in their results and did not include premature infants in the lower GA range who commonly survive nowadays. Marks and Gross[42] found higher activity in preterm infants than term infants of the same postnatal age, but their analysis pooled infants aged 2 days to 1 year. Stewart and Birkbeck[43] did report premature infant G6PD activity higher than in term infants, and term infants were correspondingly higher than adults, while decreasing GA correlated inversely with G6PD activity. Herz and colleagues[44] documented higher G6PD activity in low BW infants 865 to 2160 g, but pooled preterm and term neonates. Oski and colleagues[45] found higher G6PD activity in preterms compared with adults, but not significantly higher than in term infants.

Mesner and colleagues[46] performed a broad study of 94 Israeli, male preterm infants from 23 to 36 weeks gestation and compared them with term infants 37 weeks GA or older. Overall, for those in the normal range, G6PD activity in the premature infant group was significantly higher than in the term infants (14.2 ± 4.6 versus 12.0 ± 3.8 U/g Hb, respectively, $P = .03$). Further analysis demonstrated that the increased activity was limited to the premature group in the 29- to 32-week GA group, whereas those less than 29 or greater than 32 weeks GA were similar to the 37-week or older GA group (**Fig. 3**).

Ko and colleagues[47] in Hong Kong confirmed overall higher G6PD activity in preterm infants (GA 30.7 ± 0.3 weeks GA) compared with term counterparts (13.52 ± 0.19 versus 12.36 ± 0.16 U/g Hb, $P<.001$). In contrast to the findings of Mesner and colleagues,[46] they found progressively increasing enzyme activity as GA decreased. However, the differences between preterm and term infants may have been muted, and the effect of decreasing GA modified, by the inclusion of

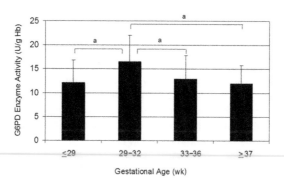

Fig. 3. G6PD activity (mean $\pm$ SD) for the 3 subgroups of premature infants and the term and near term neonates. [a] $P<.001$. (*From* Mesner O, Hammerman C, Goldschmidt D, et al. Glucose-6-phosphate dehydrogenase activity in male premature and term neonates. Arch Dis Child Fetal Neonatal Ed 2004;89:F556; with permission.)

heterozygotes in their analysis, the result of pooling equal numbers of female and male newborns in both patient groups.

Glucose-6-Phosphate Dehydrogenase-Deficient Premature Infants

Despite the increased activity level in term infants adequate for G6PD, in male infants, there should be no difficulty in diagnosing G6PD deficiency in the affected infants.[39,41] Similarly, 4 of the premature infants in the study by Mesner and colleagues[46] were clearly G6PD-deficient with low G6PD activity (all $\leq$1.8 U/g Hb), and with no overlap with the G6PD-adequate group. Female infants, on the other hand, may be more difficult to diagnose by biochemical means because many may be heterozygotes with nonrandom X chromosome inactivation, and therefore, a wide range of G6PD activity. Biochemical methods may accurately designate the phenotype in G6PD-deficient or normal homozygotes, but may be only suggestive of heterozygosity.[30] Molecular technology is the only way of accurately designating G6PD genotype in the female infant.

PREVENTION AND TREATMENT OF HYPERBILIRUBINEMIA IN PRETERM, GLUCOSE-6-PHOSPHATE DEHYDROGENASE-DEFICIENT NEWBORNS
Prevention

The prevention of bilirubin neurotoxicity in these infants may be accomplished, at least in part, by avoidance of known triggers of hemolysis and early recognition of jaundice (hyperbilirubinemia) in those in whom it is developing, in order to facilitate institution of treatment with phototherapy or exchange transfusion, if possible, before the onset of bilirubin encephalopathy. In this respect, some G6PD-deficient preterm infants may be at an advantage in that they remain under close observation, in hospital, and within a premature unit. Development of hyperbilirubinemia may therefore be detected in its early stages and its progression halted by appropriate therapy. Not so for the late preterm infant who is often discharged within a few days of delivery and is now dependent primarily on the parents, and sometimes community health care workers, to identify rapidly evolving hyperbilirubinemia.

Treatment

Extreme hyperbilirubinemia
Preterm neonates with extreme hyperbilirubinemia, or with signs of ABE, should be managed by a "crash-cart approach."[4] Intensive phototherapy should be instituted while blood is being set up for exchange transfusion, or during transport to a center capable of doing the exchange, and exchange transfusion performed as soon as feasible.

Moderate hyperbilirubinemia
Preterm infants with moderate hyperbilirubinemia should be managed according to the American Academy of Pediatrics 2004 guideline,[48] using the lower TB indications (preterm plus risk factors) for phototherapy and exchange transfusion.

An approach to the prevention and treatment of G6PD deficiency associated neonatal hyperbilirubinemia is summarized in **Box 4**.[49]

Neonatal Screening for Glucose-6-Phosphate Dehydrogenase Deficiency

In 1989, the Working Committee of the World Health Organization (WHO) recommended that neonatal screening for G6PD deficiency be performed in population groups with a male incidence of greater than 3% to 5%.[7] The aim of screening is to identify newborns at high risk for developing hyperbilirubinemia so as to facilitate timely

---

Box 4
Suggested approach to prevention and treatment of glucose-6-phosphate dehydrogenase deficiency associated neonatal hyperbilirubinemia

1. Population screening of newborn babies in populations with a frequency of G6PD deficiency greater than 3% to 5% (WHO Working Group recommendations). This can be expanded to universal screening in geographic areas with nonhomogenous population groups.

2. Combine screening program with education campaign for parents and health care workers. Specifically, parents should be warned to avoid eating or cooking fava beans in their homes, especially during breast-feeding. Clothes from a previous baby, which had been stored in naphthalene-containing mothballs, should not be used. Sulpha-containing antimicrobials should be avoided, as should triple dye or menthol-containing umbilical potions. Henna, used by some population groups to color the skin, should be scrupulously avoided.

3. Vigilant monitoring for development of jaundice both at home and in community clinics

4. Aggressive institution of therapy
   a. Intensive phototherapy
   b. Exchange transfusion

From Kaplan M, Hammerman C, Bhutani VK. Parental education and the WHO neonatal G-6-PD screening program: a quarter century later. J Perinatol 2015;35:780; with permission.

---

approach to medical facilities and the institution of therapy. Education of parents and community workers is integral to any screening program, both as to which foods and chemical substances to avoid and also as to recognize the development of jaundice, or deepening of jaundice, in those in whom it already is apparent. Despite these recommendations, neonatal screening for G6PD deficiency has not been adopted universally. In those countries in which it has been instituted, screening in combination with parental education has been instrumental in diminishing the incidence of bilirubin encephalopathy and kernicterus, as recently reviewed.[49] In the United States, G6PD screening has been instituted in a limited fashion only.[50]

G6PD screening should not be regarded as unnecessary in the preterm infant. Even within the relatively protected environment of a premature unit, hyperbilirubinemia may occur, and extreme hyperbilirubinemia may develop within days of discharge, as illustrated in the cases above.

PRETERM INFANTS REQUIRING BLOOD OR EXCHANGE TRANSFUSION

It is not routine practice to screen healthy blood donors for G6PD deficiency. Case reports have identified transfusion of G6PD-deficient RBCs as causing hemolysis and other adverse events, as summarized by Francis and colleagues.[51] In preterm infants, 2 newborns had episodes of hemolysis following blood transfusion.[52] The only anomaly found that could explain the hemolysis in these infants was that the donors were G6PD-deficient, whereas the infants had normal G6PD activity. These investigators suggest that screening for G6PD deficiency may be necessary before blood is transfused to a preterm infant. Kumar and colleagues[53] describe a 34-week GA infant who developed acute hemolysis following exchange transfusion with blood from a G6PD-deficient donor. Samanta and colleagues[54] compared 21 newborns who had undergone exchange transfusion with G6PD-deficient blood with 114 in whom G6PD-normal blood was used. The mean GA of the infants in both groups was in the late preterm range. Although the percentage decrease in TB immediately after the exchange was similar in both groups, during the following days the difference became less marked in those who had been exchanged with G6PD-deficient blood. Similarly, the mean duration of phototherapy and number of newborns that required repeat exchange transfusion were higher in the recipients of G6PD-deficient blood. The investigators attribute these effects to hemolysis of the G6PD-deficient RBCs following the exchange transfusion.

Although WHO guidelines suggest that blood from G6PD-deficient donors without a known history of hemolysis may be used for general purposes, it does suggest that its use is not acceptable for intrauterine transfusions, for neonatal transfusions, or in G6PD-deficient patients.[55] US and UK blood transfusion guidelines do not offer strategies for G6PD screening or use of G6PD-deficient blood.[56,57] Francis and colleagues[51] calculated that approximately 45,000 units of G6PD-deficient blood are transfused annually in the United States, making it not unlikely that a preterm infant will receive an affected blood transfusion. The suggested mechanism of the hemolysis is that patients requiring RBC transfusions may be simultaneously receiving oxidative medications or have concurrent infections, both of which can induce hemolysis in the G6PD-deficient RBCs. Christensen and colleagues[58] have demonstrated an increase in TB following blood transfusion (not necessarily with G6PD-deficient blood) in preterm infants. It stands to reason that the preterm, with inherent immaturity of the bilirubin conjugation system, will be at greater risk than more mature counterparts should he be transfused with G6PD-deficient blood with the potential of hemolysis.

Should Preterm Infants Receive Only Glucose-6-Phosphate Dehydrogenase-Normal Blood?

In a meta-analysis, Renzaho and colleagues[59] conclude that, in general, for adult recipients, the risks of transfusion with G6PD-deficient blood are minimal. They do suggest, however, that for preterm infants or neonates requiring exchange transfusion, G6PD screening of the donor blood may be appropriate.

SUMMARY AND BEST PRACTICES

- G6PD deficiency is commonly occurring with a worldwide distribution.
- The condition is associated with acute hemolysis, often, but not exclusively, due to an identifiable trigger, with resultant extreme hyperbilirubinemia and its consequence of bilirubin neurotoxicity.
- By virtue of shortened RBC lifespan in combination with diminished bilirubin conjugative ability, the preterm infant is inherently at high risk for hemolysis and severe hyperbilirubinemia. Smaller preterm infants may be at an advantage in that they remain hospitalized and under observation for the immediate postnatal period. Late preterm infants are often discharged along with their term counterparts and may develop hyperbilirubinemia of sudden and acute onset while at home.
- G6PD screening with parental education as to which foodstuffs and chemical substances to avoid and how to identify developing jaundice should facilitate the timely approach to medical facilities before the onset of bilirubin encephalopathy.
- Screening of donor blood for use in preterm infants for G6PD deficiency should be considered when the potential for transfusing G6PD-deficient blood is high.

REFERENCES

1. Beutler E. G6PD deficiency [Review]. Blood 1994;84:3613–36.
2. Cappellini MD, Fiorelli G. Glucose-6-phosphate dehydrogenase deficiency. Lancet 2008;371:64–74.

3. Olusanya BO, Emokpae AA, Zamora TG, et al. Addressing the burden of neonatal hyperbilirubinaemia in countries with significant glucose-6-phosphate dehydrogenase deficiency. Acta Paediatr 2014;103:1102–9.
4. Johnson L, Bhutani VK, Karp K, et al. Clinical report from the pilot USA Kernicterus Registry (1992 to 2004). J Perinatol 2009;29(Suppl 1):S25–45.
5. Sgro M, Campbell D, Shah V. Incidence and causes of severe neonatal hyperbilirubinemia in Canada. CMAJ 2006;175:587–90.
6. Manning D, Todd P, Maxwell M, et al. Prospective surveillance study of severe hyperbilirubinaemia in the newborn in the UK and Ireland. Arch Dis Child Fetal Neonatal Ed 2007;92:F342–6.
7. Glucose-6-phosphate dehydrogenase deficiency. WHO Working Group. Bull World Health Organ 1989;67:601–11.
8. Chinevere TD, Murray CK, Grant E Jr, et al. Prevalence of glucose-6-phosphate dehydrogenase deficiency in U.S. Army personnel. Mil Med 2006;171:905–7.
9. Kaplan M, Vreman HJ, Hammerman C, et al. Favism by proxy in nursing glucose-6-phosphate dehydrogenase-deficient neonates. J Perinatol 1998;18(6 Pt 1):477–9.
10. Kaplan M, Hammerman C. Glucose-6-phosphate dehydrogenase deficiency and severe neonatal hyperbilirubinemia: a complexity of interactions between genes and environment. Semin Fetal Neonatal Med 2010;15:148–56.
11. Kaplan M, Hammerman C, Vreman HJ, et al. Severe hemolysis with normal blood count in a glucose-6-phosphate dehydrogenase deficient neonate. J Perinatol 2008;28:306–9.
12. Kaplan M, Vreman HJ, Hammerman C, et al. Contribution of haemolysis to jaundice in Sephardic Jewish glucose-6-phosphate dehydrogenase deficient neonates. Br J Haematol 1996;93:822–7.
13. Kaplan M, Rubaltelli FF, Hammerman C, et al. Conjugated bilirubin in neonates with glucose-6-phosphate dehydrogenase deficiency. J Pediatr 1996;128(5 Pt 1):695–7.
14. Kaplan M, Renbaum P, Levy-Lahad E, et al. Gilbert syndrome and glucose-6-phosphate dehydrogenase deficiency: a dose-dependent genetic interaction crucial to neonatal hyperbilirubinemia. Proc Natl Acad Sci U S A 1997;94:12128–32.
15. Kawade N, Onishi S. The prenatal and postnatal development of UDP-glucuronyltransferase activity towards bilirubin and the effect of premature birth on this activity in the human liver. Biochem J 1981;196:257–60.
16. Watchko JF, Maisels MJ. The enigma of low bilirubin kernicterus in premature infants: why does it still occur, and is it preventable? Semin Perinatol 2014;38:397–406.
17. Kaplan M, Bromiker R, Hammerman C. Hyperbilirubinemia, hemolysis, and increased bilirubin neurotoxicity. Semin Perinatol 2014;38:429–37.
18. Watchko JF. Hyperbilirubinemia and bilirubin toxicity in the late preterm infant. Clin Perinatol 2006;33:839–52.
19. Kaplan M, Herschel M, Hammerman C, et al. Neonatal hyperbilirubinemia in African American males: the importance of glucose-6-phosphate dehydrogenase deficiency. J Pediatr 2006;149:83–8.
20. Zangen S, Kidron D, Gelbart T, et al. Fatal kernicterus in a girl deficient in glucose-6-phosphate dehydrogenase: a paradigm of synergistic heterozygosity. J Pediatr 2009;154:616–9.
21. Beutler E, Gelbart T, Demina A. Racial variability in the UDP-glucuronosyltransferase 1 (UGT1A1) promoter: a balanced polymorphism

for regulation of bilirubin metabolism? Proc Natl Acad Sci U S A 1998;95: 8170–4.

22. Kaplan M, Slusher T, Renbaum P, et al. (TA)n UDP-glucuronosyltransferase 1A1 promoter polymorphism in Nigerian neonates. Pediatr Res 2008;63:109–11.

23. Kaplan M, Muraca M, Hammerman C, et al. Imbalance between production and conjugation of bilirubin: a fundamental concept in the mechanism of neonatal jaundice. Pediatrics 2002;110:e47.

24. Kaplan M, Muraca M, Vreman HJ, et al. Neonatal bilirubin production-conjugation imbalance: effect of glucose-6-phosphate dehydrogenase deficiency and borderline prematurity. Arch Dis Child Fetal Neonatal Ed 2005; 90:F123–7.

25. Kaplan M, Hammerman C, Renbaum P, et al. Differing pathogenesis of perinatal bilirubinemia in glucose-6-phosphate dehydrogenase-deficient versus-normal neonates. Pediatr Res 2001;50:532–7.

26. Eshaghpour E, Oski FA, Williams M. The relationship of erythrocyte glucose-6-phosphate dehydrogenase deficiency to hyperbilirubinemia in Negro premature infants. J Pediatr 1967;70:595–601.

27. Owa JA, Dawodu AH. Neonatal jaundice among Nigerian preterm infants. West Afr J Med 1990;9:252–7.

28. Ashkenazi S, Mimouni F, Merlob P, et al. Neonatal bilirubin levels and glucose-6-phosphate dehydrogenase deficiency in preterm and low-birth-weight infants in Israel. Isr J Med Sci 1983;19:1056–8.

29. Costa S, De Carolis MP, De Luca D, et al. Severe hyperbilirubinemia in a glucose-6-phosphate dehydrogenase-deficient preterm neonate: could prematurity be the main responsible factor? Fetal Diagn Ther 2008;24(4):440–3.

30. Meloni T, Cutillo S, Testa U, et al. Neonatal jaundice and severity of glucose-6-phosphate dehydrogenase deficiency in Sardinian babies. Early Hum Dev 1987;15:317–22.

31. Nair V, Hasan SU, Romanchuk K, et al. Bilateral cataracts associated with glucose-6-phosphate dehydrogenase deficiency. J Perinatol 2013;33:574–5.

32. Lodha A, Kamaluddeen MS, Kelly E, et al. Clostridium difficile infection precipitating hemolysis in glucose-6-phosphate dehydrogenase-deficient preterm twins causing severe neonatal jaundice. J Perinatol 2008;28:77–8.

33. Turbendian HK, Perlman JM. Glucose-6-phosphate dehydrogenase deficiency in triplets of African-American descent. J Perinatol 2006;26:201–3.

34. Shah VA, Yeo CL. Massive acute haemolysis and severe neonatal hyperbilirubinemia in glucose-6-phosphate dehydrogenase-deficient preterm triplets. J Paediatr Child Health 2007;43:411–3.

35. Tanphaichitr VS, Pung-amritt P, Yodthong S, et al. Glucose-6-phosphate dehydrogenase deficiency in the newborn: its prevalence and relation to neonatal jaundice. Southeast Asian J Trop Med Public Health 1995; 26(Suppl 1):137–41.

36. Kaplan M, Beutler E, Vreman HJ, et al. Neonatal hyperbilirubinemia in glucose-6-phosphate dehydrogenase-deficient heterozygotes. Pediatrics 1999;104(1 Pt 1): 68–74.

37. Kaplan M, Hammerman C, Vreman HJ, et al. Acute hemolysis and severe neonatal hyperbilirubinemia in glucose-6-phosphate dehydrogenase-deficient heterozygotes. J Pediatr 2001;139:137–40.

38. Luzzatto L. Glucose 6-phosphate dehydrogenase deficiency: from genotype to phenotype. Haematologica 2006;91:1303–6.

39. Algur N, Avraham I, Hammerman C, et al. Quantitative neonatal glucose-6-phosphate dehydrogenase screening: distribution, reference values, and classification by phenotype. J Pediatr 2012;161:197–200.
40. Riskin A, Gery N, Kugelman A, et al. Glucose-6-phosphate dehydrogenase deficiency and borderline deficiency: association with neonatal hyperbilirubinemia. J Pediatr 2012;161:191–6.e1.
41. Kaplan M, Hoyer JD, Herschel M, et al. Glucose-6-phosphate dehydrogenase activity in term and near-term, male African American neonates. Clin Chim Acta 2005;355:113–7.
42. Marks PA, Gross RT. Erythrocyte glucose-6-phosphate dehydrogenase deficiency: evidence of differences between Negroes and Caucasians with respect to this genetically determined trait. J Clin Invest 1959;38: 2253–62.
43. Stewart AG, Birkbeck JA. The activities of lactate dehydrogenase, transaminase, and glucose-6-phosphate dehydrogenase in the erythrocytes and plasma of newborn infants. J Pediatr 1962;61:395–404.
44. Herz F, Kaplan E, Scheye ES. A longitudinal study of red cell enzymes in infants of low birth weight. Z Kinderheilkd 1975;120:217–21.
45. Oski FA, Smith C, Brigandi E. Red cell metabolism in the premature infant. Apparent inappropriate glucose consumption for cell age. Pediatrics 1968;41: 473–82.
46. Mesner O, Hammerman C, Goldschmidt D, et al. Glucose-6-phosphate dehydrogenase activity in male premature and term neonates. Arch Dis Child Fetal Neonatal Ed 2004;89:F555–7.
47. Ko CH, Wong RP, Ng PC, et al. Oxidative challenge and glucose-6-phosphate dehydrogenase activity of preterm and term neonatal red blood cells. Neonatology 2009;96:96–101.
48. American Academy of Pediatrics Subcommittee on Hyperbilirubinemia. Management of hyperbilirubinemia in the newborn infant 35 or more weeks of gestation. Pediatrics 2004;114:297–316.
49. Kaplan M, Hammerman C, Bhutani VK. Parental education and the WHO neonatal G-6-PD screening program: a quarter century later. J Perinatol 2015; 35(10):779–84.
50. Watchko JF, Kaplan M, Stark AR, et al. Should we screen newborns for glucose-6-phosphate dehydrogenase deficiency in the United States? J Perinatol 2013; 33:499–504.
51. Francis RO, Jhang JS, Pham HP, et al. Glucose-6-phosphate dehydrogenase deficiency in transfusion medicine: the unknown risks. Vox Sang 2013;105: 271–82.
52. Mimouni F, Shohat S, Reisner SH. G6PD-deficient donor blood as a cause of hemolysis in two preterm infants. Isr J Med Sci 1986;22:120–2.
53. Kumar P, Sarkar S, Narang A. Acute intravascular haemolysis following exchange transfusion with G-6-PD deficient blood. Eur J Pediatr 1994;153:98–9.
54. Samanta S, Kumar P, Kishore SS, et al. Donor blood glucose-6-phosphate dehydrogenase deficiency reduces the efficacy of exchange transfusion in neonatal hyperbilirubinemia. Pediatrics 2009;123:e96–100.
55. Stainsby D, Dhingr N, James V, et al. Blood donor selection: guidelines on assessing donor suitability for blood donation. Geneva (Switzerland): World Health Organization; 2012.
56. American Association of Blood Banks. Standards for blood banks and transfusion services. Bethesda (MD): 28. AABB Press; 2012.

57. Blood safety and quality regulations 2005. (United Kingdom): 2005. Available at: http://www.legislation.gov.uk/uksi/2005/50/pdfs/uksi_20050050_en.pdf. Accessed February 15, 2016.

58. Christensen RD, Baer VL, Snow GL, et al. Association of neonatal red blood cell transfusion with increase in serum bilirubin. Transfusion 2014;54:3068–74.

59. Renzaho AM, Husser E, Polonsky M. Should blood donors be routinely screened for glucose-6-phosphate dehydrogenase deficiency? A systematic review of clinical studies focusing on patients transfused with glucose-6-phosphate dehydrogenase-deficient red cells. Transfus Med Rev 2014;28:7–17.

Glucose-6-Phosphate Dehydrogenase Deficiency and the Need for a Novel Treatment to Prevent Kernicterus

CrossMark

Anna D. Cunningham, BS, Sunhee Hwang, PhD,
Daria Mochly-Rosen, PhD*

KEYWORDS

- Hyperbilirubinemia • Bilirubin • Kernicterus • G6PD deficiency • Jaundice
- Neurotoxicity • Activator • Chaperone

KEY POINTS

- Glucose-6-phosphate dehydrogenase (G6PD) deficiency increases the risk of kernicterus in jaundiced newborns.
- G6PD is a major source of protection against bilirubin-induced oxidative stress in the developing brain.
- There is need in both developed and developing nations for a novel treatment for kernicterus, especially in regions with a high rate of G6PD deficiency.
- The authors propose a small-molecule activator or pharmacologic chaperone for G6PD as a therapy for kernicterus in both G6PD-deficient and -normal infants with hyperbilirubinemia.

INTRODUCTION

Approximately 80% of newborns worldwide have some degree of hyperbilirubinemia and visible jaundice.[1] Severe cases of hyperbilirubinemia can progress to kernicterus and lead to permanent developmental disorders. Several risk factors contribute to hyperbilirubinemia and kernicterus, including glucose-6-phosphate dehydrogenase (G6PD) deficiency, which is one of the most common human enzymopathies. In the developing world, lack of access to common treatments for hyperbilirubinemia, along with a high rate of G6PD deficiency, leads to a high incidence of kernicterus. In this article, the authors highlight the need for a novel therapy to prevent kernicterus and discuss the pharmacologic activation of G6PD as a promising therapeutic strategy.

Disclosure Statement: The authors have nothing to disclose.
Department of Chemical and Systems Biology, Stanford University, 269 Campus Drive, Stanford, CA 94305, USA
* Corresponding author. 269 Campus Drive, CCSR 3145, Stanford, CA 94305.
E-mail address: mochly@stanford.edu

Clin Perinatol 43 (2016) 341–354
http://dx.doi.org/10.1016/j.clp.2016.01.010   perinatology.theclinics.com
0095-5108/16/$ – see front matter © 2016 Elsevier Inc. All rights reserved.

HYPERBILIRUBINEMIA AND KERNICTERUS

Hyperbilirubinemia results from increased bilirubin production coupled with inefficient bilirubin excretion. Hemolysis and subsequent heme breakdown produce bilirubin, which is conjugated and excreted in the liver. However, an immature liver-conjugating ability in newborns leads to reduced bilirubin removal and increased levels of bilirubin in circulation.

Low to moderate levels of total serum/plasma bilirubin (TB) levels (<20 mg/dL) are nontoxic and can be reduced by noninvasive treatments such as phototherapy, which uses light in a narrow wavelength band with a peak around 460 to 490 nm to photodegrade bilirubin into excretable byproducts. In cases of severe hyperbilirubinemia, exchange transfusion is used. Other therapies, less commonly used, include intravenous immunoglobulin (mechanism of action unknown) and pharmacologic therapies to reduce bilirubin production or increase bilirubin conjugation.[2]

If severe hyperbilirubinemia is left untreated, bilirubin can cross the blood-brain barrier, leading to acute bilirubin encephalopathy, which is reversible if identified and treated early. If chronic, kernicterus can result, which is characterized by lethargy, decreased feeding, high-pitched cry, fever, seizures, and even death. Up to 84% of infants with kernicterus will develop chronic bilirubin encephalopathy, characterized by permanent movement disorders, mental retardation, and hearing loss.[3]

It is difficult to estimate the incidence of kernicterus because of delayed diagnosis, an error in the ICD coding, underreporting, or lack of reporting in third-world countries.[4] The incidence of severe hyperbilirubinemia is estimated to be 2 to 45 per 100,000 births, and of kernicterus to be 0.4 to 2.7 per 100,000 births in developed countries.[5] The incidence of kernicterus in developing countries is higher due to a variety of factors, such as poor infrastructure, lack of resources, genetic differences, prematurity, low birth weight, home birthing, underfeeding, and sepsis.[5–7]

GLUCOSE-6-PHOSPHATE DEHYDROGENASE DEFICIENCY

G6PD deficiency is one of the most common human enzymopathies and is estimated to affect 400 million people worldwide, with 11 million G6PD-deficient infants born each year.[8,9] The deficiency is caused by single-nucleotide polymorphisms (SNPs) leading to single amino acid changes in the protein. More than 400 SNPs, responsible for 160 different amino acid changes, have been observed in G6PD deficiency.[10,11] These mutations can cause deficiencies of varying severities and are classified into 4 clinical categories (Table 1). Most of the G6PD deficiencies can be accounted for by a few common and relatively mild (class II or III) mutations,

Table 1
Clinical classification of glucose-6-phosphate dehydrogenase mutations

Classification of G6PD Mutations		Clinical Outcome
Class I	<10% activity	Severe; CNSHA
Class II	<10% activity	Severe episodes of hemolytic anemia
Class III	10%–60% activity	Mild episodes of hemolytic anemia
Class IV	60%–150% activity	Asymptomatic

Adapted from Cappellini MD, Fiorelli G. Glucose-6-phosphate dehydrogenase deficiency. Lancet 2008;371:64–74.

whereas severe (class I) mutations are rare.[12] Because G6PD is X-linked, heterozygous female infants can carry severe mutations and remain symptomless, whereas hemizygous male infants with class I mutations suffer from chronic nonspherocytic hemolytic anemia (CNSHA).[13,14] Class II and III mutations can lead to episodes of hemolytic anemia after exposure to stressors, such as ingestion of fava beans (favism) or certain prescription drugs or infection.

GLUCOSE-6-PHOSPHATE DEHYDROGENASE DEFICIENCY INCREASES THE RISK OF NEONATAL HYPERBILIRUBINEMIA AND KERNICTERUS

Infants with G6PD deficiency are significantly more likely to develop hyperbilirubinemia.[15] A recent meta-analysis of 5 studies including more than 20,000 subjects found that G6PD-deficient infants are almost 4 times more likely to develop hyperbilirubinemia and 3 times more likely to receive phototherapy compared with G6PD-normal infants.[16]

Moreover, G6PD-deficient infants are more likely to develop kernicterus. In the United States, 20% of infants who develop kernicterus have G6PD deficiency, compared with an estimated 4% to 7% prevalence of G6PD deficiency in the average population.[17,18] Of infants with kernicterus, 15% of those with G6PD-deficiency died, compared with 1% mortality in the G6PD-normal infants.[18] A summary of kernicterus and G6PD deficiency in other countries is summarized in **Table 2**. Enrichment of G6PD deficiency in kernicterus is seen in almost all cases.

Interestingly, African American neonates exhibit lower peak levels of TB compared with Caucasian neonates, but are more likely to develop kernicterus after discharge from the hospital, accounting for 25% of all kernicterus cases in the United States.[19] Because G6PD deficiency is highly common in African Americans (up to 21% of male infants in certain regions), this suggests that G6PD-deficient neonates develop signs of kernicterus at lower TB levels than G6PD-normal neonates.

In many Asian, African, Mediterranean, and Middle Eastern countries, where G6PD deficiency is common, all newborns are screened for G6PD deficiency. This screening has been associated with reduction of the instance of severe hyperbilirubinemia and kernicterus in several countries. In regions where G6PD deficiency is historically less common, an increase in global population movement has raised the question of whether G6PD-deficiency screening should be implemented everywhere.[17]

HOW DOES GLUCOSE-6-PHOSPHATE DEHYDROGENASE DEFICIENCY CONTRIBUTE TO KERNICTERUS?

G6PD is the rate-limiting enzyme in the pentose phosphate pathway, catalyzing the oxidation of glucose-6-phosphate to 6-phospho-gluconate while reducing nicotinamide adenine dinucleotide phosphate ($NADP^+$) to NADPH. NADPH then fuels the regeneration of reduced glutathione (GSH), which in turn neutralizes reactive oxygen species (ROS) **(Fig. 1)**. G6PD is a major source of NADPH, along with mitochondrial enzymes, isocitrate dehydrogenase, and malic enzyme.[20] However, in erythrocytes, which lack mitochondria, G6PD is the sole source of NADPH, and therefore, plays a critical role in protection against ROS. Indeed, class I G6PD mutations cause CNSHA because of lack of protection against ROS in red blood cells (RBCs). Similarly, G6PD deficiency in infants leads to an increase in hemolysis and subsequent increase in TB levels from heme breakdown and partially explains the higher prevalence of hyperbilirubinemia in G6PD-deficient infants.

The mechanism by which G6PD deficiency contributes to kernicterus is less well understood.[21] Unconjugated bilirubin accumulates in the brain, specifically in

Table 2
Kernicterus is more than 7 times more likely to occur in glucose-6-phosphate dehydrogenase-deficient newborns worldwide

Summary of Known Kernicterus and G6PD Deficiency Rates in Various Countries

Country	Incidence of Kernicterus (per 100,000)	% G6PD Deficiency in Infants with Kernicterus	Expected % G6PD Deficiency, Based on General Population	Fold Overrepresentation of G6PD Deficiency in Infants with Kernicterus	Ref.
Canada	2.3–7.9	39–58	0–3	30 X	8,75–77
Cuba	4.6	5	2–4	1.6 X	78,79
Denmark	1.8–9	2	0–3	1 X	8,80,81
Hong Kong	269	55	3–6	12 X	82
Nigeria	800–1600	61–80	15	4.7 X	83–86
Oman	346	70	18	3.9 X	87
Singapore	N/A	43	2	22 X	88
Turkey	N/A	18	13	1.4 X	89
USA	1.5	20	1–7	5.6 X	8,18,90
UK/Ireland	0.9	21	0–3	13 X	8,91
Average	—	—	—	7.5 X	—

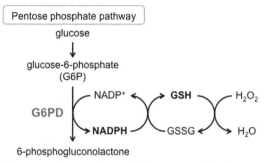

Fig. 1. Role of G6PD in protecting against oxidative stress. G6P, glucose-6-phosphate.

neurons, neuronal processes, and microglia.[22] A high rate of hemolysis may cause TB to increase more quickly than it can be conjugated or diffuse into skin and other body tissues; during this spike in which TB concentrations are higher than the diffusion threshold, bilirubin penetrates the blood-brain barrier and enters brain cells.[23] Furthermore, because bilirubin is lipophilic, it preferentially accumulates in fatty tissue, and therefore, does not diffuse out of the brain even at high brain concentrations.

Bilirubin toxicity begins at the cell membranes, because bilirubin is lipophilic and is highly concentrated in membrane compartments,[24] causing membrane permeability, leading to lipid peroxidation, and inhibiting the functions of membrane-bound proteins, such as ATPases.[25] Similarly, bilirubin also targets mitochondrial membranes, leading to disruption of the electron transport chain and membrane-bound proteins, which, in turn, results in mitochondrial swelling, membrane permeability, depolarization, cytochrome *c* release, and cell death by apoptosis and necrosis.[26–30]

Bilirubin itself has antioxidant properties, yet generation of ROS is a hallmark of bilirubin toxicity in the brain.[30–32] At high bilirubin concentrations, increased production of superoxide radical anion,[33] depletion of GSH, and increase in the oxidized disulfide form of glutathione (GSSG) are observed.[34] High concentrations of ROS lead to protein oxidation, lipid peroxidation, and DNA damage, which activates pathways signaling for neuroinflammation, cell cycle arrest, and apoptosis.[21,35] In G6PD-deficient infants, kernicterus and increased bilirubin-induced neurotoxicity can be partially attributed to the lack of GSH regeneration due to decreased G6PD activity.

In general, the brain is sensitive to damage from increased ROS because of its high utilization of oxygen and high concentration of oxidizable polyunsaturated fatty acids.[36] In addition, infants (especially preterm) have lower levels of antioxidant enzymes and scavengers such as vitamin E.[37–39] Furthermore, the developing brain exhibits very low mitochondrial antioxidant activity and relies primarily on cytoplasmic enzymes (such as G6PD) to maintain redox homeostasis.[36]

Although the mechanism of bilirubin-induced neurotoxicity is not completely understood, it is clear that G6PD deficiency contributes to kernicterus via at least 2 mechanisms: initially, through increased hemolysis-induced spike in TB levels and subsequent accumulation of bilirubin in the brain, and second, by reduced buffering capacity against bilirubin-induced ROS (**Fig. 2**). This second mechanism may explain why G6PD-deficient infants develop kernicterus even at lower levels of TB.

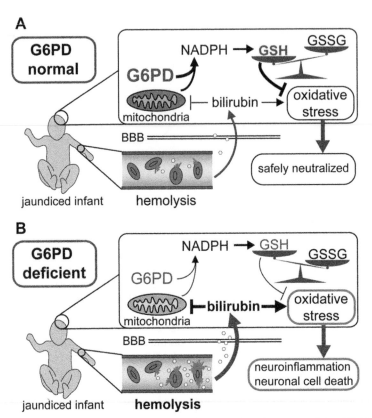

Fig. 2. Contribution of G6PD deficiency to bilirubin-induced neurotoxicity. (*A*) Neonatal hyperbilirubinemia results from production of bilirubin (*yellow hexagons*) following hemolysis. In G6PD-normal infants, GSH levels are properly maintained and low levels of bilirubin-induced oxidative stress are safely neutralized. (*B*) In G6PD-deficient infants, higher levels of hemolysis lead to higher concentration of bilirubin in the brain, which inhibits mitochondrial activity (indicated by yellowed mitochondria). Reduced G6PD activity leads to low NADPH levels, and GSH is depleted in favor of GSSG. Buildup of ROS leads to neuroinflammation, cell death, and kernicterus. BBB, blood-brain barrier.

HOW TO PREVENT KERNICTERUS?

The incidence of kernicterus has risen in recent years because of a variety of factors[5,40,41]: infants are often discharged from the hospital within 24 to 48 hours of birth, despite the fact that TB levels often peak 4 to 5 days after birth; the lack of proper monitoring at home allows the development of kernicterus, which might have otherwise been prevented if the infant were to remain at the hospital.[42] Increasing popularity of breast-feeding has also contributed to hyperbilirubinemia and kernicterus.[40,43]

In developing regions, access to phototherapy and exchange transfusions is often limited.[44] Even in developed nations, despite these simple and accessible treatments, up to 6.6% of G6PD-deficient infants will develop kernicterus,[45] and 12% to 50% of G6PD-deficient infants with kernicterus will die.[46] Especially in cases where an acute hemolytic event in G6PD-deficient infants triggers a rapid increase of bilirubin concentration in the brain, kernicterus may be impossible to prevent by conventional treatments.[47] Furthermore, exchange transfusion leads to adverse events in 5% of infants, and death in 0.4% of infants.[48]

There is a clear need for a novel therapy to prevent kernicterus and its complications, especially in G6PD-deficient newborns. In later discussion, possible approaches to treat or prevent kernicterus are proposed.

Strategies to Reduce Total Bilirubin Levels

One approach is to reduce the amount of circulating TB by increasing bilirubin conjugation, increasing the binding capacity of albumin for bilirubin, or by binding bilirubin with an exogenous therapeutic agent before it can cross the blood-brain barrier. Phenobarbital increases expression of UGT1A1, which enhances bilirubin conjugation in the liver and has been shown to reduce peak TB levels. However, the use of phenobarbital is no longer recommended due to its slow onset of effect, long duration of effect, and ineffectiveness when given in the first 12 hours of life.[49]

Previously, therapeutic attempts to increase binding of bilirubin by albumin via a small molecule have been unsuccessful.[50,51] The normal range of TB in the blood is 6 mg/dL (102 μmol/L), and at least 25 mg/dL (427 μmol/L) in cases of severe hyperbilirubinemia.[42] With this extremely high TB concentration, a therapeutic bilirubin-binding agent would need to reach an unreasonably high concentration in the blood in order to have a physiologically significant effect.

Treatment with Antioxidants

Major bilirubin toxicity stems from GSH depletion and imbalanced redox equilibrium. Although bilirubin induces upregulation of genes involved in GSH homeostasis, NADPH homeostasis, and antioxidant defense,[52,53] the temporal delay in upregulation may allow ample time for spikes in bilirubin-related ROS to exert neuronal damage. Studies have shown that levels of antioxidant vitamins A, C, and E are reduced in hyperbilirubinemic infants[54]; however, a clinical study showed that treating infants with hyperbilirubinemia with the antioxidant vitamin E was unsuccessful.[55]

A more recent study showed that total antioxidant capacity remains unchanged or may increase in hyperbilirubinemia, possibly due to the antioxidant activity of bilirubin.[56] This interplay between antioxidant activity and ROS is characteristic of other ROS-related diseases, and although bilirubin-induced ROS is a main driver of kernicterus, the use of antioxidants to prevent kernicterus is likely to be ineffective. Antioxidant treatment has proven ineffective in many other ROS-related diseases,[57,58] possibly because these antioxidants may be scavenging both good and bad ROS.[59] Furthermore, the transient, spikelike nature of bilirubin-induced ROS is difficult to pinpoint, and administration of antioxidants too early or too late will not be effective.

Therefore, restoring redox equilibrium by improving endogenous antioxidant defense represents a more promising treatment for kernicterus and ROS-related diseases in general.

Restoring Endogenous Glutathione: Activating Glucose-6-Phosphate Dehydrogenase

Specifically, GSH depletion and increase in GSSG are hallmarks of bilirubin toxicity; a therapy directed at restoring the GSH/GSSG balance may be more helpful than general treatment with antioxidants. For example, pretreatment with N-acetylcysteine (NAC), a GSH precursor, reduced bilirubin toxicity in rat neuronal cells in culture.[34,52] NAC has been administered to preterm infants with no ill effects, but its effect on development of hyperbilirubinemia and/or kernicterus has not been reported.[60] However, supplementing with GSH or GSH precursors does not bypass the issue of timing, and sudden increase in GSH may have unwanted impacts on glucose and/or iron metabolism.[58,61] Moreover, GSH does not efficiently cross the blood-brain barrier,[62] and it is unknown whether NAC can cross the blood-brain barrier.[63] Rather, a therapy directed at maintaining endogenous control of the GSH/GSSG balance is desirable.

G6PD is the rate-limiting producer of cytoplasmic NADPH, which in turn converts GSSG to GSH (see **Fig. 1**). As discussed, in the developing brain, mitochondrial production of NADPH is low and is made even lower by the toxic effect of bilirubin on the mitochondrial membrane. Therefore, G6PD is the main driver of GSH regeneration. The loss of this major source of GSH in G6PD deficiency explains why higher rates and worse outcomes of kernicterus are observed in G6PD-deficient infants. Therefore, the authors propose a small-molecule activator or chaperone of G6PD as a novel treatment for kernicterus. Discovery of molecular chaperones and activators is uncommon compared with the discovery of small-molecule enzyme inhibitors, but a few small-molecule chaperones have been used successfully.

One example is a pharmacologic chaperone therapy for Gaucher disease, a lysosomal storage disease. The disease is caused by mutations in acid β-glucosidase leading to significant protein misfolding and subsequent degradation of the protein before it can be transported to the lysosome. Interestingly, binding of small molecule inhibitors to the mutated protein rescues protein folding and allows the protein to be transported to the lysosome; these inhibitors have been termed "pharmacologic chaperones." The pharmacologic chaperone is competitively replaced by the highly concentrated substrate in the lysosome, leading to a net gain in acid β-glucosidase activity. Pharmacologic chaperones have entered phase II clinical trials to treat Gaucher disease in humans.[64]

Several common G6PD variants, such as G6PD A⁻, which is present in up to 45% of the population in some regions of Africa,[8] and G6PD Mediterranean, which is the most common G6PD mutation in Caucasians,[65] have been found to exhibit misfolding[66,67] and reduced half-life in RBCs.[68] Moreover, many class I G6PD mutations exhibit highly decreased thermostability[69] and inefficient protein folding.[70] A pharmacologic chaperone similar to the one found for Gaucher disease may be an effective strategy for correcting these types of G6PD mutations (**Fig. 3A**).

Another example of a small-molecule activator is Alda-1, an activator of aldehyde dehydrogenase 2 (ALDH2). A common ALDH2 variant, referred to as ALDH2*2, shows disordered folding in a small region of the protein caused by a single amino acid mutation. The ALDH2*2 variant remains viable, but exhibits less than 5% activity of ALDH2. Alda-1 increases the activity of ALDH2*2 by 11-fold and allosterically restores folding to the disordered region as demonstrated by a cocrystal structure.[71,72] Moreover, Alda-1 also increases the activity of wild-type ALDH2 by 2-fold. Crystallography shows that Alda-1 binds near the active site, increasing productive encounters between the substrate and catalytic residues.[71]

Most G6PD mutants have not been crystallized, but if mutations induce disordered regions similar to ALDH2*2, they could potentially be corrected allosterically by a small molecule in a mechanism similar to Alda-1 (**Fig. 3B**). Canton G6PD, the most common mutation in East Asia, has been crystallized but shows no gross structural differences compared with wild-type G6PD.[73,74] In this case, a small molecule activator could be identified that binds in the catalytic site of G6PD and

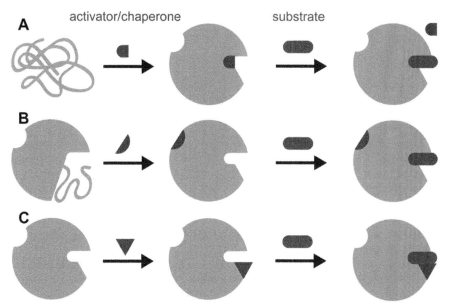

Fig. 3. Mechanisms of pharmacologic chaperone or small-molecule activator. (*A*) A pharmacologic chaperone rescues misfolding. In the case of pharmacologic chaperones for acid β-glucosidase, the chaperone is competitively replaced by substrate. (*B*) A small molecule activator correcting a disordered region allosterically. (*C*) A small molecule activator binding in the active site, increasing productive interaction between substrate and catalytic residues.

facilitates substrate and/or cofactor binding (**Fig. 3**C). Such a small molecule could also potentially activate wild-type G6PD in the same fashion; this activator could serve as a treatment to prevent kernicterus even in G6PD-normal infants with hyperbilirubinemia.

Best practices

What is the current practice?

- Jaundiced infants with TB levels greater than 20 mg/dL are subjected to phototherapy and generally are given exchange transfusion at the TB level greater than 25 mg/dL.

- Phototherapy and exchange transfusion may not be available in developing nations where G6PD deficiency is most common.

What changes in current practice are likely to improve outcomes?

- The authors propose development of a novel treatment to prevent kernicterus in addition to current practice.

- A G6PD activator or pharmacologic chaperone may reduce hemolysis and increase protection against bilirubin-induced ROS in the developing brain.

- Screening for G6PD deficiency even in regions where G6PD deficiency is uncommon may help identify infants at higher risk for developing kernicterus.

Summary Statement

Preventable kernicterus and the subsequent long-term sequelae still occur with regular frequency in both developed and developing nations. The authors propose activation of G6PD as a novel treatment for kernicterus in both G6PD-deficient and G6PD-normal infants.

REFERENCES

1. Maisels MJ. Managing the jaundiced newborn: a persistent challenge. CMAJ 2015;187:335–43.
2. Watchko JF, Tiribelli C. Bilirubin-induced neurologic damage—mechanisms and management approaches. N Engl J Med 2013;369:2021–30.
3. Kaplan M, Hammerman C. Understanding severe hyperbilirubinemia and preventing kernicterus: adjuncts in the interpretation of neonatal serum bilirubin. Clin Chim Acta 2005;356:9–21.
4. Bhutani VK, Johnson LH, Jeffrey Maisels M, et al. Kernicterus: epidemiological strategies for its prevention through systems-based approaches. J Perinatol 2004;24:650–62.
5. Olusanya BO, Ogunlesi TA, Slusher TM. Why is kernicterus still a major cause of death and disability in low-income and middle-income countries? Arch Dis Child 2014;99:1117–21.
6. Bhutani VK, Wong RJ. Bilirubin neurotoxicity in preterm infants: risk and prevention. J Clin Neonatol 2013;2:61–9.
7. Arain YH, Bhutani VK. Prevention of kernicterus in South Asia: role of neonatal G6PD deficiency and its identification. Indian J Pediatr 2014;81:599–607.
8. Nkhoma ET, Poole C, Vannappagari V, et al. The global prevalence of glucose-6-phosphate dehydrogenase deficiency: a systematic review and meta-analysis. Blood Cells Mol Dis 2009;42:267–78.
9. Bhutani VK, Zipursky A, Blencowe H, et al. Neonatal hyperbilirubinemia and Rhesus disease of the newborn: incidence and impairment estimates for 2010 at regional and global levels. Pediatr Res 2013;74:86–100.
10. Beutler E. G6PD: population genetics and clinical manifestations. Blood Rev 1996;10:45–52.
11. Minucci A, Moradkhani K, Hwang MJ, et al. Glucose-6-phosphate dehydrogenase (G6PD) mutations database: review of the "old" and update of the new mutations. Blood Cells Mol Dis 2012;48:154–65.
12. Cappellini MD, Fiorelli G. Glucose-6-phosphate dehydrogenase deficiency. Lancet 2008;371:64–74.
13. Luzzatto L. Glucose 6-phosphate dehydrogenase deficiency: from genotype to phenotype. Haematologica 2006;91:1303–6.
14. Corrons JV, Feliu E, Pujades MA, et al. Severe-glucose-6-phosphate dehydrogenase (G6PD) deficiency associated with chronic hemolytic anemia, granulocyte dysfunction, and increased susceptibility to infections: description of a new molecular variant (G6PD Barcelona). Blood 1982;59:428–34.
15. Kaplan M, Hammerman C. Glucose-6-phosphate dehydrogenase deficiency and severe neonatal hyperbilirubinemia: a complexity of interactions between genes and environment. Semin Fetal Neonatal Med 2010;15:148–56.
16. Liu H, Liu W, Tang X, et al. Association between G6PD deficiency and hyperbilirubinemia in neonates: a meta-analysis. Pediatr Hematol Oncol 2015;32:92–8.
17. Watchko JF, Kaplan M, Stark AR, et al. Should we screen newborns for glucose-6-phosphate dehydrogenase deficiency in the United States? J Perinatol 2013;33:499–504.
18. Johnson L, Bhutani VK, Karp K, et al. Clinical report from the pilot USA kernicterus registry (1992 to 2004). J Perinatol 2009;29(Suppl 1):S25–45.
19. Watchko JF. Hyperbilirubinemia in African American neonates: clinical issues and current challenges. Semin Fetal Neonatal Med 2010;15:176–82.

20. Tomanek L. Proteomic responses to environmentally induced oxidative stress. J Exp Biol 2015;218:1867–79.
21. Brites D, Brito MA. Bilirubin toxicity. In: Stevenson DK, Maisels MJ, Watchko JF, editors. Care of the jaundiced neonate. New York: The McGraw-Hill Companies, Inc; 2012. p. 115–43.
22. Martich-Kriss V, Kollias SS, Ball WS. MR findings in kernicterus. AJNR Am J Neuroradiol 1995;16:819–21.
23. Kaplan M, Bromiker R, Hammerman C. Hyperbilirubinemia, hemolysis, and increased bilirubin neurotoxicity. Semin Perinatol 2014;38:429–37.
24. Hansen T, Tommarello S, Allen J. Subcellular localization of bilirubin in rat brain after in vivo i.v. administration of [3H]bilirubin. Pediatr Res 2001;49:203–7.
25. Brito MA, Brites D, Butterfield DA. A link between hyperbilirubinemia, oxidative stress and injury to neocortical synaptosomes. Brain Res 2004;1026:33–43.
26. Rodrigues CM, Solá S, Castro RE, et al. Perturbation of membrane dynamics in nerve cells as an early event during bilirubin-induced apoptosis. J Lipid Res 2002;43:885–94.
27. Keshavan P, Schwemberger SJ, Smith DL, et al. Unconjugated bilirubin induces apoptosis in colon cancer cells by triggering mitochondrial depolarization. Int J Cancer 2004;112:433–45.
28. Rodrigues CM, Solá S, Silva R, et al. Bilirubin and amyloid-beta peptide induce cytochrome c release through mitochondrial membrane permeabilization. Mol Med 2000;6:936–46.
29. Rodrigues CM, Solá S, Brites D. Bilirubin induces apoptosis via the mitochondrial pathway in developing rat brain neurons. Hepatology 2002;35:1186–95.
30. Oakes GH, Bend JR. Early steps in bilirubin-mediated apoptosis in murine hepatoma (Hepa 1c1c7) cells are characterized by aryl hydrocarbon receptor-independent oxidative stress and activation of the mitochondrial pathway. J Biochem Mol Toxicol 2005;19:244–55.
31. Seubert JM, Darmon AJ, El-Kadi AO, et al. Apoptosis in murine hepatoma hepa 1c1c7 wild-type, C12, and C4 cells mediated by bilirubin. Mol Pharmacol 2002; 62:257–64.
32. Cesaratto L, Calligaris SD, Vascotto C, et al. Bilirubin-induced cell toxicity involves PTEN activation through an APE1/Ref-1-dependent pathway. J Mol Med 2007;85:1099–112.
33. Loftspring MC, Johnson HL, Feng R, et al. Unconjugated bilirubin contributes to early inflammation and edema after intracerebral hemorrhage. J Cereb Blood Flow Metab 2011;31:1133–42.
34. Vaz AR, Silva SL, Barateiro A, et al. Selective vulnerability of rat brain regions to unconjugated bilirubin. Mol Cell Neurosci 2011;48:82–93.
35. Hsieh H-L, Yang C-M. Role of redox signaling in neuroinflammation and neurode-generative diseases. Biomed Res Int 2013;2013:e484613.
36. Ikonomidou C, Kaindl AM. Neuronal death and oxidative stress in the developing brain. Antioxid Redox Signal 2010;14:1535–50.
37. Lindeman JH, van Zoeren-Grobben D, Schrijver J, et al. The total free radical trapping ability of cord blood plasma in preterm and term babies. Pediatr Res 1989;26:20–4.
38. Sullivan JL, Newton RB. Serum antioxidant activity in neonates. Arch Dis Child 1988;63:748–50.
39. McElroy MC, Postle AD, Kelly FJ. Catalase, superoxide dismutase and glutathione peroxidase activities of lung and liver during human development. Biochim Biophys Acta 1992;1117:153–8.

40. Watchko JF. Identification of neonates at risk for hazardous hyperbilirubinemia: emerging clinical insights. Pediatr Clin North Am 2009;56:671–87.
41. Ives K. Preventing kernicterus: a wake-up call. Arch Dis Child Fetal Neonatal Ed 2007;92:F330–1.
42. Bhutani VK, Johnson L. Kernicterus in the 21st century: frequently asked questions. J Perinatol 2009;29:S20–4.
43. Gourley GR. Breast-feeding, neonatal jaundice and kernicterus. Semin Neonatol 2002;7:135–41.
44. Olusanya BO, Slusher TM. Reducing the burden of severe neonatal jaundice in G6PD-deficient populations in low-income countries: are we doing enough? Int Health 2010;2:22–4.
45. Weng Y-H, Chiu Y-W. Clinical characteristics of G6PD deficiency in infants with marked hyperbilirubinemia. J Pediatr Hematol Oncol 2010;32:11–4.
46. Kaplan M, Bromiker R, Hammerman C. Severe neonatal hyperbilirubinemia and kernicterus: are these still problems in the third millennium? Neonatology 2011; 100:354–62.
47. Kaplan M, Hammerman C. Glucose-6-phosphate dehydrogenase deficiency: a hidden risk for kernicterus. Semin Perinatol 2004;28:356–64.
48. Muchowski KE. Evaluation and treatment of neonatal hyperbilirubinemia. Am Fam Physician 2014;89:873–8.
49. American Academy of Pediatrics. Management of hyperbilirubinemia in the newborn infant 35 or more weeks of gestation. Pediatrics 2004;114:297–316.
50. Woods JT, Bryan LE, Chan G, et al. Gentamicin and albumin-bilirubin binding. An in vivo study. J Pediatr 1976;89:483–6.
51. Brossard Y, Larsen M, Mesnard G, et al. Bilirubin-albumin-binding function of 2 human albumin preparations (placental and plasma). Comparison of their efficacy in the icteric premature infant. Arch Fr Pédiatr 1988;45:91–7 [in French].
52. Qaisiya M, Coda Zabetta CD, Bellarosa C, et al. Bilirubin mediated oxidative stress involves antioxidant response activation via Nrf2 pathway. Cell Signal 2014;26:512–20.
53. Deganuto M, Cesaratto L, Bellarosa C, et al. A proteomic approach to the bilirubin-induced toxicity in neuronal cells reveals a protective function of DJ-1 protein. Proteomics 2010;10:1645–57.
54. Turgut M, Başaran O, Çekmen M, et al. Oxidant and antioxidant levels in preterm newborns with idiopathic hyperbilirubinaemia. J Paediatr Child Health 2004;40: 633–7.
55. Fischer AF, Inguillo D, Martin DM, et al. Carboxyhemoglobin concentration as an index of bilirubin production in neonates with birth weights less than 1,500 grams: a randomized double-blind comparison of supplemental oral vitamin E and placebo. J Pediatr Gastroenterol Nutr 1987;6:748–51.
56. Bélanger S, Lavoie JC, Chessex P. Influence of bilirubin on the antioxidant capacity of plasma in newborn infants. Biol Neonate 1997;71:233–8.
57. Guallar E, Stranges S, Mulrow C, et al. Enough is enough: stop wasting money on vitamin and mineral supplements. Ann Intern Med 2013;159:850–1.
58. Kawagishi H, Finkel T. Unraveling the truth about antioxidants: ROS and disease: finding the right balance. Nat Med 2014;20:711–3.
59. Carocho M, Ferreira IC. A review on antioxidants, prooxidants and related controversy: natural and synthetic compounds, screening and analysis methodologies and future perspectives. Food Chem Toxicol 2013;51:15–25.
60. Soghier LM, Brion LP. Cysteine, cystine or N-acetylcysteine supplementation in parenterally fed neonates. Cochrane Database Syst Rev 2006;4:CD004869.

61. Kumar C, Igbaria A, D'Autreaux B, et al. Glutathione revisited: a vital function in iron metabolism and ancillary role in thiol-redox control: GSH crucial for iron metabolism, minor for redox. EMBO J 2011;30:2044–56.

62. Smeyne M, Smeyne RJ. Glutathione metabolism and Parkinson's disease. Free Radic Biol Med 2013;62:13–25.

63. Samuni Y, Goldstein S, Dean OM, et al. The chemistry and biological activities of N-acetylcysteine. Biochim Biophys Acta 2013;1830:4117–29.

64. Benito JM, Garcia Fernández JM, Mellet CO. Pharmacological chaperone therapy for Gaucher disease: a patent review. Expert Opin Ther Pat 2011;21: 885–903.

65. Oppenheim A, Jury CL, Rund D, et al. G6PD Mediterranean accounts for the high prevalence of G6PD deficiency in Kurdish Jews. Hum Genet 1993;91:293–4.

66. Gómez-Gallego F, Garrido-Pertierra A, Mason PJ, et al. Unproductive folding of the human G6PD-deficient variant A-. FASEB J 1996;10:153–8.

67. Gómez-Gallego F, Garrido-Pertierra A, Bautista JM. Structural defects underlying protein dysfunction in human glucose-6-phosphate dehydrogenase A– deficiency. J Biol Chem 2000;275:9256–62.

68. Piomelli S, Corash LM, Davenport DD, et al. In vivo lability of glucose-6-phosphate dehydrogenase in GdA- and GdMediterranean deficiency. J Clin Invest 1968;47:940–8.

69. Gómez-Manzo S, Terrón-Hernández J, De la Mora-De la Mora I, et al. The stability of G6PD is affected by mutations with different clinical phenotypes. Int J Mol Sci 2014;15:21179–201.

70. Wang X-T, Engel PC. Clinical mutants of human glucose 6-phosphate dehydrogenase: impairment of NADP(+) binding affects both folding and stability. Biochim Biophys Acta 2009;1792:804–9.

71. Perez-Miller S, Younus H, Vanam R, et al. Alda-1 is an agonist and chemical chaperone for the common human aldehyde dehydrogenase 2 variant. Nat Struct Mol Biol 2010;17:159–64.

72. Chen C-H, Budas GR, Churchill EN, et al. An activator of mutant and wildtype aldehyde dehydrogenase reduces ischemic damage to the heart. Science 2008;321:1493–5.

73. Kotaka M, Gover S, Vandeputte-Rutten L, et al. Structural studies of glucose-6-phosphate and NADP+ binding to human glucose-6-phosphate dehydrogenase. Acta Crystallogr D Biol Crystallogr 2005;61:495–504.

74. Au SW, Gover S, Lam VM, et al. Human glucose-6-phosphate dehydrogenase: the crystal structure reveals a structural NADP+ molecule and provides insights into enzyme deficiency. Structure 2000;8:293–303.

75. Sgro M. Incidence and causes of severe neonatal hyperbilirubinemia in Canada. CMAJ 2006;175:587–90.

76. Sgro M, Campbell DM, Kandasamy S, et al. Incidence of chronic bilirubin encephalopathy in Canada, 2007–2008. Pediatrics 2012;130:e886–90.

77. AlOtaibi SF, Blaser S, MacGregor DL. Neurological complications of kernicterus. Can J Neurol Sci 2005;32:311–5.

78. Henny-Harry C, Trotman H. Epidemiology of neonatal jaundice at the University Hospital of the West Indies. West Indian Med J 2012;61:37–42.

79. Monteiro WM, Val FF, Siqueira AM, et al. G6PD deficiency in Latin America: systematic review on prevalence and variants. Mem Inst Oswaldo Cruz 2014;109: 553–68.

80. Bjerre JV, Petersen JR, Ebbesen F. Surveillance of extreme hyperbilirubinaemia in Denmark. A method to identify the newborn infants. Acta Paediatr 2008;97: 1030–4.

81. Ebbesen F, Andersson C, Verder H, et al. Extreme hyperbilirubinaemia in term and near-term infants in Denmark. Acta Paediatr 2005;94:59–64.

82. Lai HC, Lai MP, Leung KS. Glucose-6-phosphate dehydrogenase deficiency in Chinese. J Clin Pathol 1968;21:44–7.

83. Battistuzzi G, Esan GJ, Fasuan FA, et al. Comparison of GdA and GdB activities in Nigerians. A study of the variation of the G6PD activity. Am J Hum Genet 1977; 29:31–6.

84. Ogunlesi TA, Ogunfowora OB. Predictors of acute bilirubin encephalopathy among Nigerian term babies with moderate-to-severe hyperbilirubinaemia. J Trop Pediatr 2011;57:80–6.

85. Williams O, Gbadero D, Edowhorhu G, et al. Glucose-6-phosphate dehydrogenase deficiency in Nigerian children. PLoS One 2013;8:e68800.

86. Owa JA, Ogunlesi TA, Ogunlesi TA. Why we are still doing so many exchange blood transfusion for neonatal jaundice in Nigeria. World J Pediatr 2009;5:51–5.

87. Nair AK, Khusaiby SMA. Kernicterus and G6PD deficiency—a case series from Oman. J Trop Pediatr 2003;49:74–7.

88. Wong Hock Boon. Singapore kernicterus—the position in 1965. J Singapore Paediatr Soc 1965;7:35–43.

89. Katar S. Glucose-6-phosphate dehydrogenase deficiency and kernicterus of South-East Anatolia. J Pediatr Hematol Oncol 2007;29:284–6.

90. Burke BL, Robbins JM, Bird TM, et al. Trends in hospitalizations for neonatal jaundice and kernicterus in the United States, 1988–2005. Pediatrics 2009;123: 524–32.

91. Manning DJ, Maxwell MJ, Todd PJ, et al. Prospective surveillance study of severe hyperbilirubinaemia in the newborn in the United Kingdom and Ireland. Arch Dis Child Fetal Neonatal Ed 2006;92:F342–6.

Cholestasis in Preterm Infants

Katie Satrom, MD[a],*, Glenn Gourley, MD[b]

KEYWORDS

- Cholestasis • Direct hyperbilirubinemia • Jaundice • Preterm infant
- Parenteral nutrition associated liver disease (PNALD) • Intestinal failure
- Short bowel syndrome (SBS) • Sepsis

KEY POINTS

- Cholestasis in the preterm population has a multifactorial etiology that is distinct from direct hyperbilirubinemia in full-term infants.
- Risk factors for cholestasis include the degree of prematurity, low birthweight, prolonged use of parenteral nutrition (PN), lack of enteral feeding, recurrent sepsis, and intestinal injury.
- The disease spectrum of PN-associated liver disease ranges from mild and reversible cholestasis to end-stage liver disease requiring transplantation; the underlying mechanism is not well-understood.
- Parenteral lipid emulsions have been implicated in the development of cholestasis; alternative lipid formulations for preventing and managing liver injury is an active area of research.
- Early enteral feedings with advancement as tolerated is currently the best way to prevent and manage cholestasis in preterm infants.

INTRODUCTION

Neonatal cholestasis, in general, refers to the accumulation of bilirubin and bile acids as a result of impaired bile flow. It is manifested by an increased conjugated bilirubin (CB) fraction, which is distinct from the more common neonatal unconjugated hyperbilirubinemia. The overall incidence of neonatal cholestasis has been estimated to be 1 in 2500 live births,[1] and it is often associated with a specific disease process that requires further evaluation.

Neonatal cholestasis in the preterm population has a different and multifactorial etiology as compared with term infants. Cholestasis occurs in approximately

Disclosures: The authors have nothing to disclose.
[a] Division of Neonatology, Department of Pediatrics, University of Minnesota, 2450 Riverside Avenue, 6th Floor, East Building, Delivery Code: 8952A, Minneapolis, MN 55454, USA; [b] Pediatric Gastroenterology, Department of Pediatrics, University of Minnesota, 2450 Riverside Avenue, 6th Floor, East Building, 8952A, Minneapolis, MN 55454, USA
* Corresponding author.
E-mail address: ksatrom@umn.edu

18% to 24% of very low birth weight (VLBW) infants ($\leq$1500 g).[2,3] Most often in preterm infants, neonatal cholestasis is related to feeding intolerance and prolonged use of parenteral nutrition (PN); however, other factors that contribute include sepsis, intestinal failure secondary to necrotizing enterocolitis (NEC), perinatal hypoxia, and the side effects of medication (**Box 1**). The degree to which each of these factors contribute to a patient's cholestasis varies by the many interrelated clinical factors.[4] Advancements in neonatal intensive care and nutrition have made it possible for younger and smaller preterm infants to survive; however, the development of cholestasis and liver failure remain a real challenge in the care of these fragile patients.

INCIDENCE

The incidence of cholestasis in preterm infants varies greatly with the degree of prematurity, birth weight, and presence of additional risk factors. A retrospective review by Christensen and colleagues[5] of 6543 infants on PN identified those at greatest risk for developing cholestasis to include patients less than 750 g birth weight, those receiving PN for longer than 100 days, and those with intestinal anomalies including NEC, gastroschisis, and jejunal atresia. Beale and colleagues[6] reported that the incidence of cholestasis in premature infants was 10% after 10 days on PN and increased to 90% with more than 3 months of PN. A recent systematic review by Lauriti and colleagues[7] of 23 studies reported a 25.5% incidence of PN-associated liver disease (PNALD) in preterm neonates. These authors also suggest that the prevalence of cholestasis in neonates related to PN or intestinal failure has not changed significantly over the past 40 years, although more recent evidence shows promising results with regard to treating and preventing cholestasis in preterm infants.

ETIOLOGY AND PATHOPHYSIOLOGY
Anatomic and Functional Immaturity

The increased incidence of cholestasis in the most premature infants is likely owing in part to the functional immaturity of the hepatobiliary system itself. Compared with full-term infants, preterm neonates are inefficient at processing bile acids. They have decreased liver uptake and synthesis of bile salts, and also diminished enterohepatic circulation, leading to biliary stasis.[8] Their total bile salt pool size is also low. The preterm liver is more susceptible to toxicity, because the solubilization of toxic bile salts via sulfation, is deficient in the developing fetus and neonate.[9] Lack of enteral feeding causes decreased gastrointestinal hormone secretion and reduced bile flow, which

---

Box 1
Risk factors for cholestasis in preterm infants

Degree of prematurity

Lack of enteral feedings

Prolonged parenteral nutrition

Intestinal injury

Sepsis/inflammation

Hypoxia

Hepatotoxic medications

then exacerbates the preterm infants' immature liver function.[10] Limited enteral nutrition can also impair intestinal integrity leading to bacterial translocation and sepsis, which causes an additional toxic hit to the underdeveloped liver.[11]

Parenteral Nutrition

The development of PN has been life saving for premature neonates. Prompt initiation of PN is necessary in low birth weight preterm infants, because early and aggressive nutrition is critical while full enteral feedings are being established. PNALD has commonly been used to describe the conjugated hyperbilirubinemia and impaired bile flow that develops in patients on prolonged PN. PNALD definitions vary, but the usual criteria include a CB of 2 mg/dL or greater while being on PN for 14 or more days.[12] Both nutrient factors from the PN itself and also host factors from the neonate play roles in the development of PNALD.

The first case of PNALD was described in 1971 in a preterm, 1000-g neonate with cholestasis and cirrhosis on autopsy.[13] The disease spectrum ranges from mild cholestasis to severe portal hypertension and end-stage liver disease requiring liver transplantation.[14,15] Despite improvements in the management of cholestasis including PN composition and safety of catheter design, PNALD comes with significant risk for hepatobiliary dysfunction that can lead to irreversible liver failure and death.[16]

The composition of PN likely plays a significant role in the development of neonatal cholestasis; however, uncertainty remains as to which formulation is best. There is a growing body of literature exploring the role of parenteral lipid emulsions in the pathogenesis of PNALD. Recent articles review the mechanisms by which soy and other plant-based lipid emulsions may contribute to the development of cholestasis. Parenteral soybean oil is the most commonly used intravenous lipid in the United States.[12] It contains phytosterols that are structurally similar to cholesterol and bile acids and have been implicated in cholestasis-related liver disease.[17] More specifically, phytosterols have been shown in animal models to activate Kupffer cell inflammation and downregulate sterol transporters, thus inciting liver injury.[18] Alternatives to soy-based parenteral lipids such as fish oil, therefore, have been explored as both treatment and preventative options for PNALD, as discussed in the management section.

Alternatively, the carbohydrate and protein components of PN have been studied with respect to their role in PNALD. Studies have been performed in preterm infants comparing different doses of macronutrients, standard versus "aggressive" dosing and advancement schedules, with respect to both dextrose and amino acid infusions.[19–21] Differences in the incidence of PNALD have not been found between groups. Evidence suggests that it is the duration and total cumulative dose of PN that is a risk for PNALD, and not the initial daily concentration, rate of advancement, or final intended daily dose.[22]

Specific amino acids themselves have also been studied. Some amino acids are hepatotoxic (methionine, phenylalanine, tyrosine, and tryptophan), whereas others (glutamine and taurine) may be protective.[23] For example, infants on long-term PN are often deficient in taurine, which is a conditional essential amino acid in neonates. Taurine also acts as a prominent bile acid conjugate and may increase bile flow.[24,25] Evidence for monitoring amino acid levels and supplementing deficiencies is equivocal, but an active area of research.

Intestinal Injury

More recently, intestinal failure-associated liver disease (IFALD) is a term that has been used in the literature to describe the multiple factors contributing to liver injury in the setting of PN, beside just the PN itself. IFALD has been defined as cholestasis and resulting biliary cirrhosis in a patient receiving PN, who has underlying intestinal disease, dysfunction, or resection, having ruled out other specific etiologies of liver injury.[12] In preterm infants, those at greatest risk of developing IFALD are those recovering from surgical NEC with the most extreme form, leading to intestinal resection and short bowel syndrome (SBS).[5,26] Even without significant bowel resection, intestinal inflammation and injury alone may contribute to liver injury and cholestasis. A mouse model of IFALD combined PN with intestinal injury, leading to liver damage, cholestasis, and Kupffer cell activation. Interestingly, neither the PN nor intestinal injury alone produced similar results, suggesting that it is the combination of or interplay between soy-based lipid emulsions and intestinal injury that lead to cholestasis.[27]

Sepsis

Infection is yet another component to the multifactorial etiology of cholestasis in premature infants. In fact, any cause of a systemic inflammatory response including congenital infection, catheter-related sepsis, bacterial overgrowth, and NEC, is closely related to the development of PNALD.[4] The preterm population is known to be especially susceptible to infection. Not only is infection often the inciting factor leading to preterm birth itself, but it is also a well-known complication of long intensive care unit hospitalizations. In addition, the preterm infant's immune system is immature and inexperienced, which makes this group of patients particularly vulnerable.[28]

Bacterial and fungal infections from sources including the bloodstream, urinary tract, lung, and abdomen are associated with the development of cholestasis.[29,30] Certain pathogens, specifically gram-negative urinary tract infections, *Pneumococcus*, and *Candida*, are more commonly linked with cholestasis.[31] In a retrospective review by Sondheimer and colleagues[31] of neonates after intestinal resection, invasive infection closely preceded the development of cholestasis in approximately 90% of the cholestatic patients compared with those without cholestasis. Another retrospective review of SBS patients reported that fewer gram-positive infections were associated with a lower peak total serum/plasma bilirubin concentration.[32] Animal studies reveal a mechanism by which the inflammatory cascade including cytokines interleukin-1 and tumor necrosis factor-α inhibit hepatocellular transporters that are important in bile production and lead to fibrosis in hepatic sinusoidal cells.[33,34] Endotoxin release from systemic infection or gut inflammation may also make the liver more susceptible to injury from future infections.[4]

Catheter-related infections are an important cause of sepsis in infants on long-term PN. Rates of central line infections have decreased with aseptic line placement techniques and strict catheter care protocols; however, the risk for recurrent sepsis remains.[35] Microorganisms can enter the catheter from the insertion site, colonization of the catheter hub, contaminated fluids, or hematogenous spread from other infection sites.[36] The most common bacteria leading to central line infections include *Enterococcus faecalis, Staphylococcus aureus, Staphylococcus epidermidis, Streptococcus viridans, Escherichia coli, Klebsiella pneumonia, Proteus mirabilis,* and *Pseudomonas aeruginosa.*[37] In the neonatal population, the most common causes of late-onset sepsis include coagulase-negative staphylococci, *S aureus* and gram-negative bacilli.[38,39] Strategies for preventing and treating line infections including lock therapies are discussed elsewhere in this paper.

Bacterial overgrowth related to changes in the intestinal microbiome is another component in the development of cholestasis. In a large series of infants and children with PNALD, intestinal bacterial overgrowth was linked to the severity of intestinal inflammation.[40] This inflammation likely impairs the intestinal barrier function leading to the absorption of small molecules across the bowel wall inciting further inflammatory pathways.[41] Overt bacterial translocation with subsequent bacteremia is another risk factor, because recurrent sepsis is associated with the development of cholestasis.[42] In a mouse model that combined intestinal injury and PN, treating animals with 4 enteral antibiotics prevented liver injury and cholestasis. In a piglet model, feeding amniotic fluid before milk led to improved intestinal barrier function thought to be related to growth and immunologic factors improving intestinal maturity.[43] This evidence suggests that restoring and maintaining intestinal integrity and the microbiome could be important components in preventing and treating cholestasis in preterm neonates. Currently, there is no evidence that supports the use of prebiotics or probiotics in the management of cholestasis in preterm infants and concern remains regarding the risk of bacterial translocation and bacteremia.

Medications

Some medications frequently used in NICUs have been associated with cholestasis. Fluconazole, for example, is used to prevent invasive fungal infections, a serious complication of premature birth. Although once per day fluconazole dosing is effective prophylaxis against *Candida* infection in VLBW infants,[44] this regimen has been associated with an increased rate of cholestasis.[45] This evidence prompted some centers to decrease the frequency of fluconazole dosing, which on retrospective review at 1 center, showed a decreased risk and severity of cholestasis in the patients who received twice weekly fluconazole compared with more frequent dosing.[46] The 2 dosing regimens were compared in a prospective, randomized control trial, which showed that both regimens significantly reduced the fungal infection rates in VLBWs compared with placebo, and both had similar cholestasis rates.[47]

Cephalosporins, ceftriaxone in particular, are known to be a hyperbilirubinemia risk factor and can cause biliary sludge in neonates. Ceftriaxone can displace bilirubin from albumin, increasing the potential toxicity of unconjugated hyperbilirubinemia and the risk of kernicterus.[48] Another concern related to cholestasis specifically, is that ceftriaxone can lead to biliary sludge owing to the precipitation of calcium ceftriaxone salts. This biliary sludge can be seen on ultrasound imaging, but is known as pseudolithiasis because it is reversible upon discontinuation of the medication.[49,50]

A retrospective review found that preterm infants with cholestasis were more likely to have received steroids in the first month after birth. In addition, these patients had more severe intraventricular hemorrhage, were more likely to have clinically significant patent ductus arteriosus, and received more blood transfusions as a group. Although steroid exposure is likely an indication of degree of illness and not a direct effect on bilirubin metabolism, more research is needed to further study the association.[23]

Other Specific Diseases

Other etiologies for cholestasis for the preterm infant include specific diseases that also occur in term infants. **Box 2** lists the broad differential diagnosis for neonatal cholestasis. Examples of extrahepatic etiologies include biliary atresia and choledochal cysts. Intrahepatic causes include idiopathic neonatal hepatitis, α-1-antitrypsin deficiency, and progressive familial intrahepatic cholestasis. Of note, patients with idiopathic neonatal hepatitis are more likely to be born prematurely or have intrauterine growth restriction.[51] **Fig. 1** outlines an approach to the management of a premature infant with cholestasis, which recommends medical management until the infant weighs more than 2 kg, before pursuing further workup of these other specific disease processes.

Box 2
Differential diagnosis for neonatal cholestasis

1. Idiopathic neonatal hepatitis
2. Infections
   Viral
      Cytomegalovirus
      Rubella
      Reovirus 3
      Adenovirus
      Coxsackie virus
      Human herpes virus 6
      Varicella zoster
      Herpes simplex
      Parvovirus
      Hepatitis B and C
      Human immunodeficiency virus
   Bacterial
      Sepsis
      Urinary tract infection
      Syphilis
      Listeriosis
      Tuberculosis
   Parasitic
      Toxoplasmosis
      Malaria
3. Bile duct anomalies
   Biliary atresia
   Choledochal cyst
   Alagille syndrome
   Nonsyndromic bile duct paucity
   Inspissated bile syndrome
   Caroli syndrome
   Choledocholithiasis
   Neonatal sclerosing cholangitis
   Spontaneous common bile duct perforation
4. Metabolic disorders
   α_1-Antitrypsin deficiency
   Galactosemia
   Glycogen storage disorder type IV
   Cystic fibrosis
   Hemochromatosis
   Tyrosinemia
   Arginase deficiency
   Zellweger's syndrome
   Dubin–Johnson syndrome
   Rotor syndrome
   Hereditary fructosemia
   Niemann–Pick disease, type C
   Gaucher disease
   Bile acid synthetic disorders
   Progressive familial intrahepatic cholestasis
      North American Indian familial cholestasis
      Aagenaes syndrome
      X-linked adrenoleukodystrophy
5. Endocrinopathies
   Hypothyroidism
   Hypopituitarism (septooptic dysplasia)

6. Chromosomal disorders
    Turner syndrome
    Trisomy 18
    Trisomy 21
    Trisomy 13
    Cat eye syndrome
    Donahue syndrome (Leprechauns)

7. Toxic
    Parenteral nutrition
    Fetal alcohol syndrome
    Drugs

8. Vascular
    Budd–Chiari syndrome
    Neonatal asphyxia
    Congestive heart failure

9. Neoplastic
    Neonatal leukemia
    Histiocytosis X
    Neuroblastoma
    Hepatoblastoma
    Erythrophagocytic lymphohistiocytosis

10. Miscellaneous
    Neonatal lupus erythematosus
    'Le foie vide' (infantile hepatic nonregenerative disorder)
    Indian childhood cirrhosis

Adapted from Venigalla S, Gourley GR. Neonatal cholestasis. Semin Perinatol 2004;28:349; with permission.

CLINICAL EVALUATION
Laboratory

An increased CB level is the earliest laboratory sign indicative of hepatic dysfunction related to PN.[52] Although direct-reacting bilirubin and CB are often used interchangeably, these 2 compounds are not identical, because the direct bilirubin fraction contains delta-bilirubin. In most pediatric studies, cholestasis is defined as a CB 2 mg/dL or greater. CB is also used for monitoring and trending purposes during the treatment of hepatobiliary disease. Serum alanine aminotransferase and aspartate aminotransferase are sensitive indicators of hepatocellular injury, but they lack specificity or prognostic value.[53] Gamma-glutamyl transpeptidase (GGT) is a biliary epithelium enzyme, which is useful as an indicator of biliary tract dysfunction. It is a sensitive marker of obstructive hepatic disorders, and it helpful in distinguishing liver and bone etiologies with an elevated alkaline phosphatase, because GGT remains normal in bone disorders.[54] Late signs of hepatic dysfunction include hypoalbuminemia, prolonged coagulation, and thrombocytopenia.[55]

Triglyceride monitoring is used in clinical practice to evaluate for lipid overload related to PNALD.[56] Preterm infants have decreased function of the enzyme lipoprotein lipase owing to their decreased fat and muscle mass, and are therefore at risk of hypertriglyceridemia.[57–59] According to the recommendations of the European Society for Clinical Nutrition and Metabolism/European Society of Paediatric Gastroenterology, Hepatology and Nutrition, the parenteral lipid emulsion dose should be restricted when the serum triglyceride level reaches greater than 250 mg/dL.[59]

362

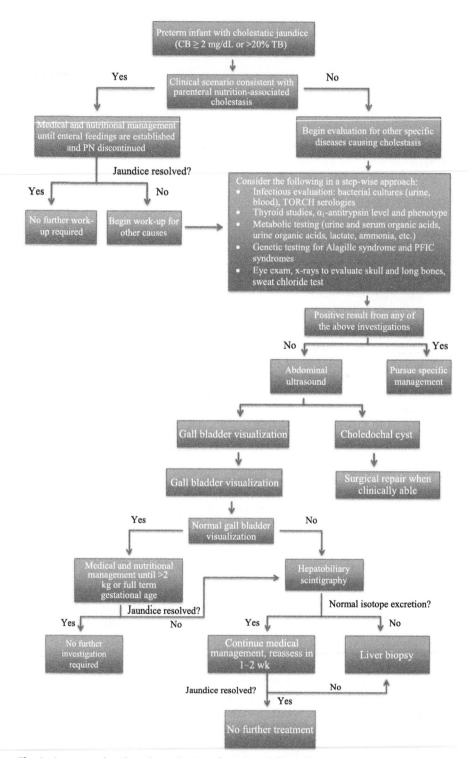

Fig. 1. A suggested guide to the evaluation of a preterm infant with cholestasis. CB, conjugated bilirubin; PFIC, progressive familial intrahepatic cholestasis; PN, parenteral nutrition; TB, total serum/plasma bilirubin; TORCH, toxoplasma, rubella, cytomegalovirus, herpes viruses. (*Adapted from* Venigalla S, Gourley GR. Neonatal cholestasis. Semin Perinatol 2004;28:350; with permission.)

Radiologic

Abdominal ultrasonography is a simple, noninvasive tool that is helpful in the workup of cholestatic infants. It can provide useful information with respect to the size and appearance of the liver and gallbladder, visualization of gallstones and sludge, and diagnosis of choledochal cysts.[60] The appropriate timing and interpretation of findings in preterm infants may be different compared with term newborns. In PNALD, ultrasound imaging of the liver and spleen could reveal nonspecific hepatomegaly, a contracted gallbladder, biliary sludge, and splenomegaly if portal hypertension exists.[55] Gallbladder length, which can be helpful in the diagnosis of biliary atresia, is small in premature infants with cholestasis.[61] The triangular cord sign, which is a more specific finding in biliary atresia, represents a fibrous cone of tissue at the porta hepatis. Although highly specific and sensitive for biliary atresia, it can be seen in any condition leading to periportal infiltration and edema, including PNALD.[62] Timing for abdominal ultrasonography in a preterm infant depends on the individual patient's clinical picture. If the history and physical examination are consistent with PNALD, then an ultrasound examination is not necessarily indicated, although it can be useful in the identification of other causes of cholestasis (eg, choledochal cyst). If the timing or degree of conjugated hyperbilirubinemia suggests an alternate etiology, then an ultrasound examination is a simple first step in the investigation.

Hepatobiliary scintigraphy and MR cholangiography are additional radiologic studies to pursue if cholestasis persists with a normal liver ultrasound examination, including gallbladder visualization. Hepatobiliary scintigraphy evaluates the patency of the biliary tract by monitoring the excretion of a technetium labeled iminodiacetic acid derivative.[63] Delayed excretion indicates possible biliary atresia or intrahepatic cholestasis. MR cholangiography is a newer technique used in neonatal imaging that has shown to be highly sensitive and specific for biliary atresia in term infants,[64] but its use has not been established in preterm infants. **Fig. 1** is a suggested evaluation guide that includes when to pursue various imaging modalities.

Liver Biopsy

Percutaneous liver biopsy is the most definitive test in the workup of neonatal cholestasis. In a premature infant, a biopsy should be postponed until the infant weighs more than 2 kg and well enough to undergo this invasive procedure. Canalicular cholestasis is the first histologic sign of PNALD, can be seen as early as 5 days after the initiation of PN in preterm infant and progresses to intracellular cholestasis after 2 weeks, then to bile duct proliferation and fibrosis after 8 weeks of PN.[65] Biopsy is indicated when the patient has continued cholestatic jaundice despite medical management and other tests are not diagnostic.

MANAGEMENT
Medical

Ursodeoxycholic acid

Ursodeoxycholic acid (UDCA) is a choleretic, hydrophilic bile acid that is not metabolized to toxic secondary bile acids, and is therefore more benign than primary human bile acids. Thus, by promoting bile flow in a nontoxic manner, it may be helpful to prevent or treat cholestasis. It is used commonly in the NICU for infants with direct hyperbilirubinemia; however, the data for UDCA in the very preterm population are limited. To our knowledge, studies to date comparing UDCA with controls are small and retrospective, with conflicting results. A study by Chen and colleagues[66] comparing 18 VLBW infants with PNALD who were treated with UDCA compared with 12 infants in the untreated control group demonstrated a shorter duration of cholestasis in the treatment group. A larger, more recent retrospective study by Thibault and colleagues[67] did not demonstrate the effect of UDCA on duration of cholestasis, however the treatment group was significantly smaller and more preterm, which is a major limitation of the study.

Cholecystokinin

Cholecystokinin is naturally released in response to a meal and promotes intrahepatic bile flow and gallbladder emptying. A synthetic analogue has been used and studied as a way to decrease gallbladder stasis and promote bile flow. There were initially positive results from small case series for its use in the prevention and treatment of PNALD in neonates.[68,69] A multicenter, randomized, controlled trial of 243 infants that compared cholecystokinin with saline, did not show any differences in either CB levels, time to enteral feeding, sepsis risk, or mortality.[70] It is therefore not recommended in the management of premature infants with cholestasis.

Erythromycin

Erythromycin has been used in the management of neonatal cholestasis to improve gastroduodenal motility and enteral feeding tolerance. A randomized controlled trial of 182 VLBW infants compared erythromycin with placebo in patients who had not yet reached one-half of full volume feedings by day of life 14. The infants who received erythromycin had a significantly lesser incidence of PNALD, shorter time to achieve full enteral feedings, and fewer episodes of sepsis.[71] This study supports the use of erythromycin in preterm infants with significant feeding intolerance as a way to promote enteral feeding and prevent PNALD.

Nutritional

Enteral nutrition

Early enteral feedings are thought to be the most important factor in preventing cholestasis in the preterm population.[72] Through limiting exposure to PN, maintaining intestinal integrity, promoting healthy immune responses, and decreasing the risk of bacterial translocation, enteral feedings help to normalize hepatobiliary function.[73] Animal studies show that lack of enteral feeding can lead to intestinal atrophy, including shortened villi and reduced enzyme activity, which are reversed with enteral feedings.[74] A randomized controlled study in preterm infants compared those receiving trophic feedings on day of life 3 and those who received only PN.[75] The infants in the trophic feeding group reached full enteral nutrition earlier, had significantly fewer episodes of culture-proven sepsis, and were discharged home sooner. There was not, however, a difference in liver function, including total serum/plasma bilirubin levels. Another randomized controlled study in growth restricted premature infants compared the early initiation of enteral feedings (on day 2) compared with delayed initiation (day 6). Infants who were fed sooner achieved full enteral feedings earlier, required fewer days of PN, had a lesser incidence of cholestatic jaundice, and trended toward fewer episodes of sepsis.[76]

Cycling parenteral nutrition

PN cycling is an approach commonly used to manage PNALD whereby a daily volume of PN is infused over a shorter period of time, which then allows 4 to 6 hours per day without PN. Data are mixed as to whether this strategy decreases the incidence of cholestasis. A retrospective study of patients with gastroschisis compared continuous PN infusion with patients who were prophylactically cycled. After adjusting for confounding factors, the group who received standard continuous infusions was more likely to develop cholestasis, but this only trended toward a statistically significant difference.[77] A randomized controlled trial in VLBW preterm infants, however, did not find that early prophylactic PN cycling reduced the incidence of cholestasis.[78] Cycling PN should be done with care, especially in the premature population, because they are at risk for hypoglycemia and other metabolic derangements, owing to insufficient nutrient stores.[22]

Lipid dose reduction
Reducing the soybean lipid emulsion dose is a commonly used strategy in the management of cholestasis in preterm infants, although the evidence behind this approach is inconclusive. A prospective cohort of surgical infants comparing those who received a reduced dose of soy-based emulsion (1 g/kg) with historical controls who received 2 to 3 g/kg, showed an almost 50% decrease in the incidence of cholestasis in the low dose group.[79] A multicenter, randomized, controlled trial in preterm neonates, however, did not find any difference in the development of cholestasis in those who received low-dose versus standard dose soy-based lipid emulsions.[80] Limiting lipid nutrition is a concern in preterm neonates, because fat is essential for normal brain growth and proper neurodevelopment.[12,81]

Alternative parenteral lipids
The use of alternative sources of parenteral lipids is currently an active area of research in the treatment and prevention of cholestasis in preterm infants. Fish oil emulsions have shown promising results in being able to reverse cholestasis.[82] Omegaven is a parenteral fish oil formulation that was initially studied in adult patients in Germany. The first US trial in infants compared 18 patients with SBS and PNALD against historical controls, and showed that Omegaven led to faster resolution of cholestasis.[83] An open-label trial produced similar results in 42 infants who received Omegaven and experience a 6-fold faster reduction in cholestasis compared with the 49 infants receiving soybean oil. The Omegaven group also had significantly fewer deaths and liver transplants.[84] Importantly, Omegaven was intended for use with other parenteral lipids in combination, not as monotherapy. Fish oil emulsions are not currently licensed for use in the United States, and are only available in investigational settings for compassionate use.[12]

There are several limitations to studies comparing soy- and fish oil-based lipid emulsions. Regarding dosage, a low-dose (1 g/kg) fish oil preparation is often compared with the standard (2–3 g/kg) soy emulsion dose. Also, fish oil emulsions contain far more α-tocopherol (vitamin E), which may itself play a role, as discussed elsewhere in this paper. These studies do not take into account long-term neurodevelopmental outcomes; using alterative or low-dose parenteral lipids may adversely affect cognitive function. A study in piglets comparing low-dose soy and fish oil emulsions compared with normal dose soy parenteral lipids revealed lower brain weight and altered brain polyunsaturated fatty acid content in the reduced dose piglets.[85] Before these new clinical practices can be adopted safely, high-quality, prospective, controlled clinical trials that include long-term neurodevelopmental outcomes are needed comparing similar doses of various lipid emulsions.

Enteral fish oil
Because the use of parenteral fish oil lacks approval by the US Food and Drug Administration, enteral fish oil is being investigated as a therapy. A murine model reported that enteral fish oil supplementation was more effective at protecting against fatty liver disease than intravenous fish oil emulsion.[86] It is thought that enteral fats induce intestinal adaptation, which is especially important in infants who underwent bowel resection.[87,88] Small case series have been published that report the resolution of PNALD in

some former preterm patients with the use of enteral fish oil. One series discontinued the soybean parenteral emulsion altogether[89] and another series continued the standard parenteral lipid in addition to enteral fish oil supplement.[72] A more recent randomized controlled trial studied early enteral fat and fish oil supplementation in premature infants who had an enterostomy. This study found that early enteral fat and fish oil administration was associated with a decreased need for intravenous lipid emulsion, improved enteral feeding, and reduced CB levels.[90] The treatment group also experienced fewer sepsis evaluations, fewer days on antibiotics, and shorter central venous line duration. There is a current randomized controlled trial underway comparing enteral fish oil with UDCA and placebo for the treatment of cholestasis in infants, with an expected completion date of April 2017 (clinicaltrials.gov).

Vitamin E

Vitamin E, specifically α-tocopherol, is a lipid-soluble antioxidant and has been implicated as a protectant against PN-associated liver toxicity. Because α-tocopherol protects unsaturated fatty acid chains from oxidative stress, it is added to lipid emulsions to prevent peroxidation.[91] It is abundant in fish oil, so the studies that provide evidence for the benefits of fish oil emulsions in the development of cholestasis, may actually point toward vitamin E as the protectant. One study in preterm piglets looked at the roles of phytosterols and vitamin E in the development of PNALD by adding phytosterols to Omegaven and α-tocopherol to soy-based parenteral emulsion. This study showed that preterm pigs that were fed PN lipid emulsions with higher vitamin E content, both soy- and fish oil-based, had lower total serum/plasma bilirubin, GGT, and serum bile acid levels compared with the standard soy-based lipid emulsions.[92] Also, this model did not demonstrate any hepatotoxicity in the pigs given phytosterols plus Omegaven, suggesting that α-tocopherol protects against damage caused by phytosterols.

Catheter Locks

Strategies in the treatment and prevention of catheter-related infections include ethanol and antibiotic lock solutions. An observational case series of pediatric oncology patients showed that ethanol locks used in addition to systemic antibiotic therapy during an acute central line infection reduced the rate of recurrence compared with patients who were only treated with antibiotics.[93] Two studies compared the rate of line infections before and after ethanol lock prophylaxis, and found that this intervention decreased the incidence of line infections from 10 per 1000 catheter-days to 2 per 1000 catheter-days.[94,95]

A recent Cochrane review evaluated 3 neonatal studies including 271 infants looking at the use of antibiotic locks in the prevention of central line infections.[96] Despite the small number of trials and different antibiotics, the use of antibiotic locks seems to be safe and effective in preventing catheter-related infection.[97,98] The risk of antibiotic resistance remains, although none of the studies showed evidence of this adverse effect. Of note, none of these studies included patients with gastrointestinal conditions or premature infants less than 28 weeks gestational age, so further research is needed to specifically study the effect of catheter locks in preterm infants.

Multidisciplinary Rehabilitation

Multidisciplinary care teams including medical, surgical, and nutritional support have been suggested to improve outcomes in neonates with PNALD. The data are heterogeneous with regard to definitions of diagnoses, study design, and patient populations; however, intestinal rehabilitation programs seem to improve mortality risk in patients with SBS.[99–101] It makes sense that a unified team of experts with consistent protocols may improve clinical outcomes. Future research is needed to not only assess mortality risk, but neurodevelopmental, quality of life, and economic outcomes as well. Protocols established at multidisciplinary rehabilitation centers could be shared with other health care systems that do not have access to such programs.[42]

Organ Transplantation

With proper, multidisciplinary management of neonatal cholestasis, the percent of children with PNALD progressing to end-stage liver disease can be decreased from its previous incidence of 10% in the 1990s to as low as 3% currently.[102] However, once an infant or child has reached the most severe stage of liver failure, mortality is high if they are not able to receive a transplant or achieve enteral independence.[103] Transplant organ donors are limited for premature infants. At 1 center, in 2001, the 10-year survival rate was 46% for intestinal transplant patients and 42% for the liver–intestine combination.[104]

Best practices

What is the current practice?

To minimize the development of cholestasis in preterm infants current practices include:
- Cautious and delayed enteral feeding;
- PN lipid dose reduction;
- PN cycling; and
- UDCA.

Best Practice Recommendation
- Early enteral feeding with advancement as clinically tolerated.
- Minimize exposure to PN without nutritional compromise.
- Aggressive sepsis prevention measures.

What changes in current practice are likely to improve outcomes

- Research regarding fish oil PN emulsions (enteral and parenteral) shows promise to decrease cholestasis in preterm infants.

- Methods to restore and maintain intestinal integrity and a healthy microbiome could be important components in preventing cholestasis in preterm neonates.

Is there a clinical algorithm?

- See **Fig. 1** for evaluation algorithm.

Summary statement

Cholestasis in preterm infants is related to multiple factors including the degree of prematurity, lack of enteral feeding, prolonged use of PN, recurrent sepsis, and intestinal injury. The development of NEC leading to bowel resection and SBS brings the greatest risk for irreversible liver failure requiring organ transplantation. Other preterm infants have more benign feeding intolerance related to intestinal immaturity and bowel dysmotility. Sepsis and inflammation from bacterial overgrowth can cause direct liver injury as well as cholestasis from decreased hepatic transporters. The composition of PN, specifically the soy-based lipid emulsions, also likely plays a role in the development of PNALD in preterm infants, and new fish oil-based solutions are being studied in the prevention and treatment of cholestasis. Evaluation of cholestasis in preterm infants starts with the monitoring of CB as well as other laboratory markers including GGT. A liver ultrasound is a first-line imaging modality that is useful in evaluating for other specific diseases causing cholestasis. Medical and nutritional therapies have been studied with mixed success in the management of cholestasis in preterm infants. Early enteral feeding, when able, is ultimately the best way to prevent and treat cholestasis in this population.

SUMMARY AND DISCUSSION

Cholestasis in preterm infants is related to multiple factors including the degree of prematurity, lack of enteral feeding, prolonged use of PN, recurrent sepsis, and intestinal injury. The development of NEC leading to bowel resection and SBS brings the greatest risk for irreversible liver failure requiring organ transplantation. Other preterm infants have more benign feeding intolerance related to intestinal immaturity and bowel dysmotility. Sepsis and inflammation from bacterial overgrowth can cause direct liver injury as well as cholestasis from decreased hepatic transporters. The composition of PN, specifically the soy-based lipid emulsions, also likely plays a role in the development of PNALD in preterm infants, and new fish oil-based solutions are being studied in the prevention and treatment of cholestasis. Evaluation of cholestasis in preterm infants starts with the monitoring of CB as well as other laboratory markers including GGT. An ultrasound examination of the liver is a first-line imaging modality that is useful in evaluating for other specific diseases causing cholestasis. Medical and nutritional therapies have been studied with mixed success in the management of cholestasis in preterm infants. Early enteral feeding, when able, is ultimately the best way to prevent and treat cholestasis in this population.

REFERENCES

1. McLin VA, Balistreri WF. Approach to neonatal cholestasis. In: Walker WA, Goulet OJ, Kleinman R, et al, editors. Pediatric gastrointestinal disease: pathophysiology, diagnosis, management. 3rd edition. Ontario (Canada): B.C. Decker, Inc; 2004. p. 1079–93.
2. Alkharfy TM, Ba-Abbad R, Hadi A, et al. Total parenteral nutrition-associated cholestasis and risk factors in preterm infants. Saudi J Gastroenterol 2014;20: 293–6.
3. Hsieh MH, Pai W, Tseng HI, et al. Parenteral nutrition-associated cholestasis in premature babies: risk factors and predictors. Pediatr Neonatol 2009;50:202–7.
4. Kaufman SS. Prevention of parenteral nutrition-associated liver disease in children. Pediatr Transplant 2002;6:37–42.
5. Christensen RD, Henry E, Wiedmeier SE, et al. Identifying patients, on the first day of life, at high-risk of developing parenteral nutrition-associated liver disease. J Perinatol 2007;27:284–90.
6. Beale EF, Nelson RM, Bucciarelli RL, et al. Intra-hepatic cholestasis associated with parenteral-nutrition in premature-infants. Pediatrics 1979;64:342–7.
7. Lauriti G, Zani A, Aufieri R, et al. Incidence, prevention, and treatment of parenteral nutrition-associated cholestasis and intestinal failure-associated liver disease in infants and children: a systematic review. JPEN J Parenter Enteral Nutr 2014;38: 70–85.
8. Watkins JB, Szczepanik P, Gould JB, et al. bile-salt metabolism in human premature-infant - preliminary observations of pool size and synthesis rate following prenatal administration of dexamethasone and phenobarbital. Gastroenterology 1975;69:706–13.
9. Watkins JB. Placental transport - bile-acid conjugation and sulfation in the fetus. J Pediatr Gastroenterol Nutr 1983;2:365–73.
10. Tyson JE, Kennedy KA. Trophic feedings for parenterally fed infants. Cochrane Database Syst Rev 2005;(3):CD0000504.
11. Takagi K, Yamamori H, Toyoda Y, et al. Modulating effects of the feeding route on stress response and endotoxin translocation in severely stressed patients receiving thoracic esophagectomy. Nutrition 2000;16:355–60.

12. Lee WS, Sokol RJ. Intestinal microbiota, lipids, and the pathogenesis of intestinal failure-associated liver disease. J Pediatr 2015;167:519–26.

13. Peden VH, Witzleben CL, Skelton MA. Total parenteral nutrition. J Pediatr 1971; 78:180–1.

14. Freund HR. Abnormalities of liver function and hepatic damage associated with total parenteral nutrition. Nutrition 1991;7:1–5 [discussion: 5–6].

15. Chan S, McCowen KC, Bistrian BR, et al. Incidence, prognosis, and etiology of end-stage liver disease in patients receiving home total parenteral nutrition. Surgery 1999;126:28–34.

16. Btaiche IF, Khalidi N. Parenteral nutrition-associated liver complications in children. Pharmacotherapy 2002;22:188–211.

17. Xu Z, Harvey KA, Pavlina T, et al. Steroidal compounds in commercial parenteral lipid emulsions. Nutrients 2012;4:904–21.

18. El Kasmi KC, Anderson AL, Devereaux MW, et al. Phytosterols promote liver injury and Kupffer cell activation in parenteral nutrition-associated liver disease. Sci Transl Med 2013;5:206ra137.

19. Wilson DC, Cairns P, Halliday HL, et al. Randomised controlled trial of an aggressive nutritional regimen in sick very low birthweight infants. Arch Dis Child Fetal Neonatal Ed 1997;77:F4–11.

20. Clark RH, Chace DH, Spitzer AR, Pediatrix Amino Acid Study Group. Effects of two different doses of amino acid supplementation on growth and blood amino acid levels in premature neonates admitted to the neonatal intensive care unit: a randomized, controlled trial. Pediatrics 2007;120:1286–96.

21. Blau J, Sridhar S, Mathieson S, et al. Effects of protein/nonprotein caloric intake on parenteral nutrition associated cholestasis in premature infants weighing 600-1000 grams. JPEN J Parenter Enteral Nutr 2007;31:487–90.

22. Rangel SJ, Calkins CM, Cowles RA, et al. Parenteral nutrition-associated cholestasis: an American Pediatric Surgical Association Outcomes and Clinical Trials Committee Systematic review. J Pediatr Surg 2012;47:225–40.

23. Steinbach M, Clark RH, Kelleher AS, et al. Demographic and nutritional factors associated with prolonged cholestatic jaundice in the premature infant. J Perinatol 2008;28:129–35.

24. Rigo J, Senterre J. Is taurine essential for the neonates? Biol Neonate 1977; 32:73–6.

25. Cooke RJ, Whitington PF, Kelts D. Effect of taurine supplementation on hepatic function during short-term parenteral nutrition in the premature infant. J Pediatr Gastroenterol Nutr 1984;3:234–8.

26. Robinson DT, Ehrenkranz RA. Parenteral nutrition-associated cholestasis in small for gestational age infants. J Pediatr 2008;152:59–62.

27. El Kasmi KC, Anderson AL, Devereaux MW, et al. Toll-like receptor 4-dependent Kupffer cell activation and liver injury in a novel mouse model of parenteral nutrition and intestinal injury. Hepatology 2012;55:1518–28.

28. Kapur R, Yoder MC, Polin RA. The immune system. In: Fanaroff A, Martin R, editors. Neonatal - perinatal medicine diseases of the fetus and infant. 9th edition. St Louis (MO): Elsevier; 2011. p. 761–93.

29. Wolf A, Pohlandt F. Bacterial infection: the main cause of acute cholestasis in newborn infants receiving short-term parenteral nutrition. J Pediatr Gastroenterol Nutr 1989;8:297–303.

30. Shamir R, Maayan-Metzger A, Bujanover Y, et al. Liver enzyme abnormalities in gram-negative bacteremia of premature infants. Pediatr Infect Dis J 2000;19: 495–8.

31. Sondheimer JM, Asturias E, Cadnapaphornchai M. Infection and cholestasis in neonates with intestinal resection and long-term parenteral nutrition. J Pediatr Gastroenterol Nutr 1998;27:131–7.

32. Andorsky DJ, Lund DP, Lillehei CW, et al. Nutritional and other postoperative management of neonates with short bowel syndrome correlates with clinical outcomes. J Pediatr 2001;139:27–33.

33. Harry D, Anand R, Holt S, et al. Increased sensitivity to endotoxemia in the bile duct-ligated cirrhotic Rat. Hepatology 1999;30:1198–205.

34. Lee JM, Trauner M, Soroka CJ, et al. Expression of the bile salt export pump is maintained after chronic cholestasis in the rat. Gastroenterology 2000;118:163–72.

35. Kelly DA. Intestinal failure-associated liver disease: what do we know today? Gastroenterology 2006;130(2 Suppl 1):S70–7.

36. Mermel LA, Farr BM, Sherertz RJ, et al. Guidelines for the management of intravascular catheter-related infections. Clin Infect Dis 2001;32:1249–72.

37. Ryder MA. Catheter-related infections: it's all about biofilm. Medsc Top Adv Pract Nurs 2005;5:1–6.

38. de Brito CS, de Brito DV, Abdallah VO, et al. Occurrence of bloodstream infection with different types of central vascular catheter in critically neonates. J Infect 2010;60:128–32.

39. O'Grady NP, Alexander M, Dellinger EP, et al. Guidelines for the prevention of intravascular catheter-related infections. Centers for Disease Control and Prevention. MMWR Recomm Rep 2002;51(RR-10):1–29.

40. Kaufman SS, Loseke CA, Lupo JV, et al. Influence of bacterial overgrowth and intestinal inflammation on duration of parenteral nutrition in children with short bowel syndrome. J Pediatr 1997;131:356–61.

41. Demehri FR, Barrett M, Ralls MW, et al. Intestinal epithelial cell apoptosis and loss of barrier function in the setting of altered microbiota with enteral nutrient deprivation. Front Cell Infect Microbiol 2013;3:105.

42. Wales PW, Allen N, Worthington P, et al. A.S.P.E.N. clinical guidelines: support of pediatric patients with intestinal failure at risk of parenteral nutrition-associated liver disease. JPEN J Parenter Enteral Nutr 2014;38:538–57.

43. Ostergaard MV, Shen RL, Stoy AC, et al. Provision of amniotic fluid during parenteral nutrition increases weight gain with limited effects on gut structure, function, immunity, and microbiology in newborn preterm pigs. JPEN J Parenter Enteral Nutr 2015. [Epub ahead of print].

44. Clerihew L, Austin N, McGuire W. Prophylactic systemic antifungal agents to prevent mortality and morbidity in very low birth weight infants. Cochrane Database Syst Rev 2007;(4):CD003850.

45. Aghai ZH, Mudduluru M, Nakhla TA, et al. Fluconazole prophylaxis in extremely low birth weight infants: association with cholestasis. J Perinatol 2006;26:550–5.

46. Bhat V, Fojas M, Saslow JG, et al. Twice-weekly fluconazole prophylaxis in premature infants: association with cholestasis. Pediatr Int 2011;53:475–9.

47. Manzoni P, Stolfi I, Pugni L, et al. A multicenter, randomized trial of prophylactic fluconazole in preterm neonates. N Engl J Med 2007;356:2483–95.

48. Martin E, Fanconi S, Kalin P, et al. Ceftriaxone – bilirubin-albumin interactions in the neonate: an in vivo study. Eur J Pediatr 1993;152:530–4.

49. Schaad UB, Wedgwood-Krucko J, Tschaeppeler H. Reversible ceftriaxone-associated biliary pseudolithiasis in children. Lancet 1988;2:1411–3.

50. Klar A, Branski D, Akerman Y, et al. Sludge ball, pseudolithiasis, cholelithiasis and choledocholithiasis from intrauterine life to 2 years: a 13-year follow-up. J Pediatr Gastroenterol Nutr 2005;40:477–80.

51. McKiernan PJ. Neonatal cholestasis. Semin Neonatol 2002;7:153–65.

52. Beath SV, Davies P, Papadopoulou A, et al. Parenteral nutrition-related cholestasis in postsurgical neonates: multivariate analysis of risk factors. J Pediatr Surg 1996; 31:604–6.

53. Best CM, Gourley GR, Bhutani VK. Neonatal cholestasis – conjugated hyperbilirubinemia. In: Buonocore G, editor. Neonatology: a practical approach to neonatal diseases. Milan (Italy): Springer; 2012. p. 650–8.

54. Hirfanoglu IM, Unal S, Onal EE, et al. Analysis of serum gamma-glutamyl transferase levels in neonatal intensive care unit patients. J Pediatr Gastroenterol Nutr 2014;58:99–101.

55. Kelly DA. Preventing parenteral nutrition liver disease. Early Hum Dev 2010;86: 683–7.

56. Toce SS, Keenan WJ. Lipid intolerance in newborns is associated with hepatic dysfunction but not infection. Arch Pediatr Adolesc Med 1995;149:1249–53.

57. Ziegler EE, O'Donnell AM, Nelson SE, et al. Body composition of the reference fetus. Growth 1976;40:329–41.

58. Valentine CJ, Puthoff TD. Enhancing parenteral nutrition therapy for the neonate. Nutr Clin Pract 2007;22:183–93.

59. Koletzko B, Goulet O, Hunt J, et al. 1. Guidelines on paediatric parenteral nutrition of the European Society of Paediatric Gastroenterology, Hepatology and Nutrition (ESPGHAN) and the European Society for Clinical Nutrition and Metabolism (ESPEN), supported by the European Society of Paediatric Research (ESPR). J Pediatr Gastroenterol Nutr 2005;41(Suppl 2):S1–87.

60. Bates MD, Bucuvalas JC, Alonso MH, et al. Biliary atresia: pathogenesis and treatment. Semin Liver Dis 1998;18:281–93.

61. Tan Kendrick AP, Phua KB, Ooi BC, et al. Making the diagnosis of biliary atresia using the triangular cord sign and gallbladder length. Pediatr Radiol 2000;30: 69–73.

62. Lee HJ, Lee SM, Park WH, et al. Objective criteria of triangular cord sign in biliary atresia on US scans. Radiology 2003;229:395–400.

63. Abramson SJ, Treves S, Teele RL. The infant with possible biliary atresia: evaluation by ultrasound and nuclear medicine. Pediatr Radiol 1982;12:1–5.

64. Han SJ, Kim MJ, Han A, et al. Magnetic resonance cholangiography for the diagnosis of biliary atresia. J Pediatr Surg 2002;37:599–604.

65. D'Apolito O, Pianese P, Salvia G, et al. Plasma levels of conjugated bile acids in newborns after a short period of parenteral nutrition. JPEN J Parenter Enteral Nutr 2010;34:538–41.

66. Chen CY, Tsao PN, Chen HL, et al. Ursodeoxycholic acid (UDCA) therapy in very-low-birth-weight infants with parenteral nutrition-associated cholestasis. J Pediatr 2004;145:317–21.

67. Thibault M, McMahon J, Faubert G, et al. Parenteral nutrition-associated liver disease: a retrospective study of ursodeoxycholic acid use in neonates. J Pediatr Pharmacol Ther 2014;19:42–8.

68. Rintala RJ, Lindahl H, Pohjavuori M. Total parenteral nutrition-associated cholestasis in surgical neonates may be reversed by intravenous cholecystokinin: a preliminary report. J Pediatr Surg 1995;30:827–30.

69. Teitelbaum DH, Han-Markey T, Drongowski RA, et al. Use of cholecystokinin to prevent the development of parenteral nutrition-associated cholestasis. JPEN J Parenter Enteral Nutr 1997;21:100–3.

70. Teitelbaum DH, Tracy TF Jr, Aouthmany MM, et al. Use of cholecystokinin-octapeptide for the prevention of parenteral nutrition-associated cholestasis. Pediatrics 2005;115:1332–40.

71. Ng PC, Lee CH, Wong SP, et al. High-dose oral erythromycin decreased the incidence of parenteral nutrition-associated cholestasis in preterm infants. Gastroenterology 2007;132:1726–39.

72. Tillman EM, Crill CM, Black DD, et al. Enteral fish oil for treatment of parenteral nutrition-associated liver disease in six infants with short-bowel syndrome. Pharmacotherapy 2011;31:503–9.

73. Adamkin DH. Total parenteral nutrition-associated cholestasis: prematurity or amino acids? J Perinatol 2003;23:437–8.

74. Pironi L, Paganelli GM, Miglioli M, et al. Morphologic and cytoproliferative patterns of duodenal mucosa in two patients after long-term total parenteral nutrition: changes with oral refeeding and relation to intestinal resection. JPEN J Parenter Enteral Nutr 1994;18:351–4.

75. McClure RJ, Newell SJ. Randomised controlled study of clinical outcome following trophic feeding. Arch Dis Child Fetal Neonatal Ed 2000;82:F29–33.

76. Leaf A, Dorling J, Kempley S, et al. Early or delayed enteral feeding for preterm growth-restricted infants: a randomized trial. Pediatrics 2012;129:e1260–8.

77. Jensen AR, Goldin AB, Koopmeiners JS, et al. The association of cyclic parenteral nutrition and decreased incidence of cholestatic liver disease in patients with gastroschisis. J Pediatr Surg 2009;44:183–9.

78. Salvador A, Janeczko M, Porat R, et al. Randomized controlled trial of early parenteral nutrition cycling to prevent cholestasis in very low birth weight infants. J Pediatr 2012;161:229–33.e1.

79. Sanchez SE, Braun LP, Mercer LD, et al. The effect of lipid restriction on the prevention of parenteral nutrition-associated cholestasis in surgical infants. J Pediatr Surg 2013;48:573–8.

80. Levit OL, Calkins KL, Gibson LC, et al. Low-dose intravenous soybean oil emulsion for prevention of cholestasis in preterm neonates. JPEN J Parenter Enteral Nutr 2014. [Epub ahead of print].

81. Nandivada P, Carlson SJ, Cowan E, et al. Role of parenteral lipid emulsions in the preterm infant. Early Hum Dev 2013;89(Suppl 2):S45–9.

82. Park HW, Lee NM, Kim JH, et al. Parenteral fish oil-containing lipid emulsions may reverse parenteral nutrition-associated cholestasis in neonates: a systematic review and meta-analysis. J Nutr 2015;145:277–83.

83. Gura KM, Lee S, Valim C, et al. Safety and efficacy of a fish-oil-based fat emulsion in the treatment of parenteral nutrition-associated liver disease. Pediatrics 2008;121:e678–86.

84. Puder M, Valim C, Meisel JA, et al. Parenteral fish oil improves outcomes in patients with parenteral nutrition-associated liver injury. Ann Surg 2009;250:395–402.

85. Josephson J, Turner JM, Field CJ, et al. Parenteral soy oil and fish oil emulsions: impact of dose restriction on bile flow and brain size of parenteral nutrition-fed neonatal piglets. JPEN J Parenter Enteral Nutr 2015;39:677–87.

86. Alwayn IP, Gura K, Nose V, et al. Omega-3 fatty acid supplementation prevents hepatic steatosis in a murine model of nonalcoholic fatty liver disease. Pediatr Res 2005;57:445–52.

87. Kollman KA, Lien EL, Vanderhoof JA. Dietary lipids influence intestinal adaptation after massive bowel resection. J Pediatr Gastroenterol Nutr 1999;28:41–5.

88. Sukhotnik I, Mor-Vaknin N, Drongowski RA, et al. Effect of dietary fat on early morphological intestinal adaptation in a rat with short bowel syndrome. Pediatr Surg Int 2004;20:419–24.

89. Rollins MD, Scaife ER, Jackson WD, et al. Elimination of soybean lipid emulsion in parenteral nutrition and supplementation with enteral fish oil improve cholestasis in infants with short bowel syndrome. Nutr Clin Pract 2010;25:199–204.

90. Yang Q, Ayers K, Welch CD, et al. Randomized controlled trial of early enteral fat supplement and fish oil to promote intestinal adaptation in premature infants with an enterostomy. J Pediatr 2014;165:274–9.e1.

91. Traber MG. Vitamin E regulatory mechanisms. Annu Rev Nutr 2007;27:347–62.

92. Ng K, Stoll B, Chacko S, et al. Vitamin E in new-generation lipid emulsions protects against parenteral nutrition-associated liver disease in parenteral nutrition-fed preterm pigs. JPEN J Parenter Enteral Nutr 2015. [Epub ahead of print].

93. Dannenberg C, Bierbach U, Rothe A, et al. Ethanol-lock technique in the treatment of bloodstream infections in pediatric oncology patients with broviac catheter. J Pediatr Hematol Oncol 2003;25:616–21.

94. Mouw E, Chessman K, Lesher A, et al. Use of an ethanol lock to prevent catheter-related infections in children with short bowel syndrome. J Pediatr Surg 2008;43:10S25–S1029.

95. Jones BA, Hull MA, Richardson DS, et al. Efficacy of ethanol locks in reducing central venous catheter infections in pediatric patients with intestinal failure. J Pediatr Surg 2010;45:1287–93.

96. Taylor JE, Tan K, Lai NM, et al. Antibiotic lock for the prevention of catheter-related infection in neonates. Cochrane Database Syst Rev 2015;(6):CD010336.

97. Filippi L, Pezzati M, Di Amario S, et al. Fusidic acid and heparin lock solution for the prevention of catheter-related bloodstream infections in critically ill neonates: a retrospective study and a prospective, randomized trial. Pediatr Crit Care Med 2007;8:556–62.

98. Garland JS, Alex CP, Henrickson KJ, et al. A vancomycin-heparin lock solution for prevention of nosocomial bloodstream infection in critically ill neonates with peripherally inserted central venous catheters: a prospective, randomized trial. Pediatrics 2005;116:e198–205.

99. Sigalet D, Boctor D, Robertson M, et al. Improved outcomes in paediatric intestinal failure with aggressive prevention of liver disease. Eur J Pediatr Surg 2009; 19:348–53.

100. Modi BP, Langer M, Ching YA, et al. Improved survival in a multidisciplinary short bowel syndrome program. J Pediatr Surg 2008;43:20–4.

101. Diamond IR, de Silva N, Pencharz PB, et al. Neonatal short bowel syndrome outcomes after the establishment of the first Canadian multidisciplinary intestinal rehabilitation program: preliminary experience. J Pediatr Surg 2007;42: 806–11.

102. Colomb V, Dabbas-Tyan M, Taupin P, et al. Long-term outcome of children receiving home parenteral nutrition: a 20-year single-center experience in 302 patients. J Pediatr Gastroenterol Nutr 2007;44:347–53.

103. Wales PW, de Silva N, Kim JH, et al. Neonatal short bowel syndrome: a cohort study. J Pediatr Surg 2005;40:755–62.

104. Abu-Elmagd K, Reyes J, Bond G, et al. Clinical intestinal transplantation: a decade of experience at a single center. Ann Surg 2001;234:404–16 [discussion: 416–7].

Development of a Web-Based Decision Support Tool to Operationalize and Optimize Management of Hyperbilirubinemia in Preterm Infants

Jonathan P. Palma, MD, MS[a,b,*,1], Yassar H. Arain, MD[a,1]

KEYWORDS

- Clinical decision support (CDS) • Practice-based evidence
- Electronic medical record (EMR) • Premie BiliRecs (PBR) • BiliTool
- Neonatal preterm hyperbilirubinemia

KEY POINTS

- Wide practice variation exists in the management of hyperbilirubinemia in preterm infants less than 35 weeks gestational age.
- Current clinical practice recommendations are consensus based and rely on expert interpretation of evidence, but would benefit from independent validation.
- Premie BiliRecs is a new web-based, electronic medical record–clinical decision support tool for dissemination of the consensus-based preterm hyperbilirubinemia management recommendations.
- Premie BiliRecs generates practice-based evidence that can be used to optimize recommendations provided by the tool itself and could serve as a tool for prospective validation.

INTRODUCTION

In 2012, Maisels and colleagues[1] published consensus-based recommendations for the management of hyperbilirubinemia in preterm infants less than 35 weeks estimated gestational age (GA). Because there is a relative paucity of data to inform

Disclosure Statement: The authors have no relevant financial interests, activities, relationships, nor affiliations to disclose.
[a] Division of Neonatal and Developmental Medicine, Department of Pediatrics, Stanford University School of Medicine, Stanford, CA, USA; [b] Department of Clinical Informatics, Stanford Children's Health, 4100 Bohannon Drive, Menlo Park, CA 94025, USA
[1] Present Address: 750 Welch Road, Suite 315, Palo Alto, CA 94304.
* Corresponding author. 750 Welch Road, Suite 315, Palo Alto, CA 94304.
E-mail address: jpalma@stanfordchildrens.org

Clin Perinatol 43 (2016) 375–383
http://dx.doi.org/10.1016/j.clp.2016.01.009
0095-5108/16/$ – see front matter © 2016 Elsevier Inc. All rights reserved.

evidence-based guidelines, the proposed thresholds represent total serum/plasma bilirubin (TB) levels at which treatment was thought likely to do more good than harm. Before the publication of these recommendations, local practices for initiation of phototherapy and exchange transfusion in premature infants varied widely,[2–4] reflecting the uncertainty in the optimal management of these infants.

The establishment of any consensus-based clinical care recommendations is an important step that naturally leads to 2 broad challenges, each representing significant opportunity. The first is the dissemination of the recommendations and their incorporation into clinical practice; even for evidence-based guidelines, it may take years to achieve widespread adoption and practice change.[5] Second, consensus-based recommendations inherently lack evidence, but by encouraging standardization of practice, they create a foundation for evaluation of their impact on patient outcomes.

Electronic clinical decision support (CDS) tools address both of these challenges. Electronic CDS tools operate at the intersection of common clinical problems and best practice recommendations to drive practice change.[6] Additionally, as a byproduct of their use, appropriately configured electronic CDS tools can generate practice-based evidence that, in turn, can be used to optimize the recommendations provided by the tool itself. For these reasons, we developed a web-based CDS tool for the management of hyperbilirubinemia in moderately preterm infants less than 35 weeks GA that operationalizes and automates the Maisels and colleagues[1] approach, and creates a platform for refining treatment recommendations.

DEVELOPMENT OF THE CLINICAL DECISION SUPPORT TOOL
Operationalizing Consensus-Based Recommendations

In contrast with the management of hyperbilirubinemia in moderately preterm infants, sufficient evidence exists regarding management of hyperbilirubinemia in infants 35 or more weeks GA that the American Academy of Pediatrics (AAP) Subcommittee on Neonatal Hyperbilirubinemia published a clinical practice guideline in 2004.[7] This guideline references the hour-specific nomogram published by Bhutani and colleagues,[8] which enabled the recommendations to be translated into an electronic CDS tool that was adopted rapidly.[9,10]

The consensus-based TB thresholds proposed by Maisels and colleagues[1] (**Table 1**), however, are not amenable to automation in their native form; the recommended TB ranges apply both to a postmenstrual age (PMA) range, and account for the clinical uncertainty in the in management of hyperbilirubinemia within a given

| Table 1 | | |
TB thresholds for moderately preterm infants		
Postmenstrual Age (weeks plus days)	Phototherapy Threshold (TB, mg/dL)	Exchange Transfusion Threshold (TB, mg/dL)
<28 + 0/7	5–6	11–14
28 + 0/7–29 + 6/7	6–8	12–14
30 + 0/7–31 + 6/7	8–10	13–16
32 + 0/7–33 + 6/7	10–12	15–18
34 + 0/7–34 + 6/7	12–14	17–19

Abbreviation: TB, total serum/plasma bilirubin.
Adapted from Maisels MJ, Watchko JF, Bhutani VK, et al. An approach to the management of hyperbilirubinemia in the preterm infant less than 35 weeks of gestation. J Perinatol 2012;32:662; with permission.

PMA category. To help address this, Wallenstein and Bhutani[11] published clinical strategies to operationalize and contextualize the consensus-based TB threshold ranges. Although the operational thresholds address clinical uncertainty in application of the recommendations to individual patients, they do not stratify threshold TB values within PMA categories, such that the same threshold might be recommended for patients up to 2 weeks apart in PMA (**Fig. 1**).

To more fully operationalize and automate the consensus-based recommendations, we converted the proposed ranges for both phototherapy and exchange transfusion into 2 linear plots for each. First, we addressed clinical uncertainty by dividing the proposed TB threshold ranges into more and less conservative thresholds based on the work of Wallenstein and Bhutani.[11] We then used linear algebra to extrapolate TB values to the nearest tenth of a decimal for each day of PMA from 27 weeks plus 0 days through 34 weeks plus 6 days (algorithm available upon request). The resulting linear plots (**Fig. 2**) represent suggested values for intervention based on the acuity of the neonate, with lower recommended TB thresholds for considering phototherapy and preparing for exchange transfusion in higher acuity patients. Recommended thresholds at which to prepare for exchange transfusion assume that effective phototherapy is being administered.

The expert consensus-based recommendations[1] are based on PMA alone and not chronologic age. Our recommended thresholds are intended for infants greater than 48 hours of age, and lower TB thresholds should be used for initiation of phototherapy at earlier chronologic ages.[2,12] This supports both the simplicity of the recommendations (because they apply to PMA only), and aligns closely with the 48-hour threshold TB values in the AAP clinical practice guideline for 35-week GA infants.

The Clinical Decision Support Tool: "Premie BiliRecs"

The web-based CDS tool, Premie BiliRecs, requires users to input a premature infant's TB value and PMA in weeks plus days on the day the TB value was obtained (**Fig. 3**). The tool accepts both US (mg/dL) and international system (μmol/L) units as specified by the user. Input controls are in place to ensure valid data entry such that a manually

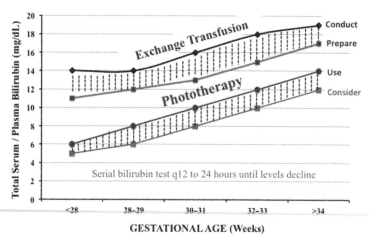

Fig. 1. Operational total serum/plasma bilirubin thresholds for moderately preterm infants. (*Adapted from* Maisels MJ, Watchko JF, Bhutani VK, et al. An approach to the management of hyperbilirubinemia in the preterm infant less than 35 weeks of gestation. J Perinatol 2012;32:660–4; with permission.)

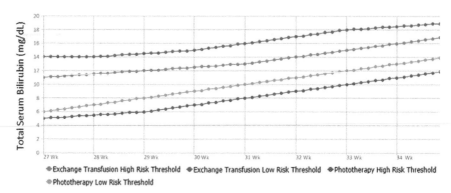

Postmenstrual Age (weeks plus days)

Fig. 2. Total serum/plasma bilirubin thresholds for moderately preterm infants ≥48 hours of age. (*Adapted from* Wallenstein MB, Bhutani VK. Jaundice and kernicterus in the moderately preterm infant. Clin Perinatol 2013;40:683; with permission.)

entered value outside the limits set for age results in a hard stop and a message about data entry limits.

The results are presented on a single response screen that includes a display of user-entered values for validation, and a table containing phototherapy and exchange transfusion recommendations (**Fig. 4**). The higher TB threshold values for phototherapy and exchange transfusion represent levels at which treatment is assumed likely to do more good than harm in patients with prematurity but no additional neurotoxicity risk factors. The lower TB threshold values for phototherapy and exchange transfusion represent levels at which it is possible that patients at higher risk for bilirubin neurotoxicity would benefit from initiation of therapy. Clinical judgment is required to determine which threshold value to use, and a list of additional neurotoxicity risk factors is displayed to aid in this determination (**Box 1**).

Process for Electronic Medical Record Integration

Integration with our electronic medical record (EMR) was achieved by creating custom logic to display a Premie BiliRecs icon exclusively for patients greater than 48 hours of age with a PMA within the range of the recommendations (27 weeks plus 0 days through 34 weeks plus 6 days) and with a recent TB level (**Fig. 5**). The icon serves as a patient-specific hyperlink that passes both the TB value and corresponding PMA to Premie BiliRecs as a part of the web address. The user immediately receives treatment recommendations on the Premie BiliRecs website without the need to enter information manually. No protected health information (eg, patient name, medical record number) is transmitted from the EMR to the website.

Select users (JP and YA) piloted Premie BiliRecs in the 40-bed, level III neonatal intensive care unit at Lucile Packard Children's Hospital at Stanford, the principal hospital within Stanford Children's Health in Stanford, California. In August 2015, EMR integration at Stanford Children's Health was achieved within our enterprise-wide commercial EMR (Epic Systems, Verona, WI). After a validation period following go-live in the neonatal intensive care unit at Lucile Packard Children's Hospital, Stanford in November 2015, Premie BiliRecs was made publically available at https://pbr.stanfordchildrens.org/ for both manual data entry and EMR integration.

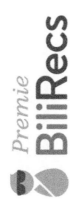

Stanford Children's Health | Lucile Packard Children's Hospital Stanford

Home   About   EMR Integration

Premie
BiliRecs

A tool for treatment of indirect hyperbilirubinemia in pre-term neonates

This tool is NOT intended for use in infants <48 hours of age.

Post-Menstrual Age: [weeks]   [days]

Total Serum Bilirubin: [mg/dl (US) ⇕]

[Submit]

Use:

Premie BiliRecs is designed to help clinicians decide when to initiate phototherapy and double volume exchange transfusion for infants < 35 weeks PMA.

Required values include the age of the child by Post-Menstrual Age, and the total bilirubin in either US (mg/dl) or SI (μmol/L) units.

Fig. 3. Premie BiliRecs data entry page. Required inputs are TB value and PMA on the day the value was obtained.

Stanford Children's Health | Lucile Packard Children's Hospital Stanford

Premie **BiliRecs**

Home   About   EMR Integration

Post-Menstrual Age: 28 weeks 6 days
Total Serum Bilirubin: 9.5 mg/dL

Additional Neurotoxicity Risk Factors

Use the lower range of the listed TSB levels for infants at greater risk for bilirubin toxicity:

1. Serum albumin levels < 2.5 g/dL
2. Rapidly rising TSB levels suggesting hemolytic disease
3. Those who are clinically unstable

Phototherapy Recommendations:

Neurotoxicity Risk Factors	TB Threshold Exceeded	Approximate TB Threshold at 28+6 Weeks Gestation
Prematurity + additional neurotoxicity risk factors	Yes	5.9 mg/dL
Prematurity alone	Yes	7.9 mg/dL

Exchange Transfusion Recommendations:

Neurotoxicity Risk Factors	TB Threshold Exceeded*	Approximate TB Threshold at 28+6 Weeks Gestation
Prematurity + additional neurotoxicity risk factors	No	11.9 mg/dL
Prematurity alone	No	14.4 mg/dL**

* Assess response to effective phototherapy

** Unable to assess neurotoxicity outcomes related to thresholds above this value

Fig. 4. Premie BiliRecs results page. Recommended TB thresholds for phototherapy and exchange transfusion.

Box 1
Preterm bilirubin neurotoxicity risk factors

1. Serum albumin levels of less than 2.5 g/dL

2. Rapidly increasing total serum/plasma bilirubin levels suggesting hemolytic disease

3. Those who are 'clinically unstable' suggested by the following:
   a. Blood pH < 7.15
   b. Blood culture positive sepsis in the prior 24 hours
   c. Apnea and bradycardia requiring cardiorespiratory resuscitation (bagging and/or intubation) during the previous 24 hours
   d. Hypotension requiring pressor treatment during the previous 24 hours
   e. Mechanical ventilation at the time of blood sampling

Limitations

The most significant limitations of Premie BiliRecs relate to the lack of available evidence to guide the management of hyperbilirubinemia in preterm infants rather than to the CDS tool itself. Preterm infants less than 27 weeks GA are theoretically more vulnerable to bilirubin toxicity than moderately preterm infants. However, owing to a lack of evidence, Premie BiliRecs does not provide recommendations for these infants until their PMA is within the range of the tool. In addition, the tool does not support recommendations for moderately preterm infants less than 48 hours of age, but obtaining TB levels is standard of care in this time period. Certainly, more conservative thresholds should be used for these newborn infants until adequate evidence exists from which to draw recommendations. It is unknown whether use of Premie BiliRecs will increase or decrease the use of phototherapy, so use of this resource should be monitored.

GENERATION OF NEW KNOWLEDGE

Perhaps the most exciting aspect of Premie BiliRecs is the opportunity to generate practice-based evidence from its routine use. In addition to the workflow benefits of EMR integration, each time the Premie BiliRecs icon is clicked, a record is created in the EMR. Because these logs exist, it is possible to retrieve patient information for premature infants treated for hyperbilirubinemia. Analyzing the outcomes of these infants will add to the evidence base available for optimization of the current consensus-based guidelines. As guidelines are updated, their incorporation into

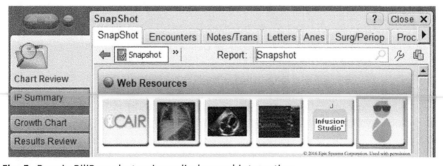

Fig. 5. Premie BiliRecs electronic medical record integration.

clinical practice can be supported through iterative updates to the recommendations provided by Premie BiliRecs. Once Premie BiliRecs is publically available for EMR integration, practice-based evidence will be generated in a variety of health care settings.

SUMMARY

Premie BiliRecs is a new, web-based CDS tool for the management of hyperbilirubinemia in moderately preterm infants less than 35 weeks GA. It operationalizes and automates current expert consensus-based guidelines,[1,11] and through EMR integration provides a platform for generation of new practice-based evidence to inform future guidelines. After local validation of the tool at Lucile Packard Children's Hospital, Premie BiliRecs will be made publically available for both manual data entry and EMR integration.

ACKNOWLEDGMENTS

The authors acknowledge and thank M. Jeffrey Maisels, Jon F. Watchko, Vinod K Bhutani, and David K. Stevenson for establishing and publishing the expert consensus guidelines that form the foundation for Premie BiliRecs, and Matthew B. Wallenstein and Vinod K. Bhutani for their work to operationalize the guidelines. Finally, we thank Joshua Faulkenberry for his technical expertise in development of the web-based CDS tool.

REFERENCES

1. Maisels MJ, Watchko JF, Bhutani VK, et al. An approach to the management of hyperbilirubinemia in the preterm infant less than 35 weeks of gestation. J Perinatol 2012;32:660–4.
2. Bratlid D, Nakstad B, Hansen TWR. National guidelines for treatment of jaundice in the newborn. Acta Paediatr 2011;100:499–505.
3. Rennie JM, Sehgal A, De A, et al. Range of UK practice regarding thresholds for phototherapy and exchange transfusion in neonatal hyperbilirubinaemia. Arch Dis Child Fetal Neonatol Ed 2009;94:F323–7.
4. Hansen TWR. Therapeutic approaches to neonatal jaundice: an international survey. Clin Pediatr 1996;35:309–16.
5. Lenfant C. Clinical research to clinical practice—lost in translation? N Engl J Med 2003;349:868–74.
6. Tierney WM. Improving clinical decisions and outcomes with information: a review. Int J Med Inform 2001;62:1–9.
7. American Academy of Pediatrics, Provisional Committee for Quality Improvement and Subcommittee on Hyperbilirubinemia. Management of hyperbilirubinemia in the newborn infant 35 or more weeks of gestation. Pediatrics 2004;114:297–316 [Erratum appears in Pediatrics 2004;114:1138].
8. Bhutani VK, Johnson L, Sivieri EM. Predictive ability of a predischarge hour-specific serum bilirubin for subsequent significant hyperbilirubinemia in healthy term and near-term newborns. Pediatrics 1999;103:6–14.
9. BiliTool. Available at: http://bilitool.org. Accessed October 10, 2015.
10. Longhurst CA, Turner S, Burgos AE. Development of a web-based decision support tool to increase use of neonatal hyperbilirubinemia guidelines. Jt Comm J Qual Patient Saf 2009;35:256–62.

11. Wallenstein MB, Bhutani VK. Jaundice and kernicterus in the moderately preterm infant. Clin Perinatol 2013;40:679–88.

12. National Institute for Health and Clinical Excellence. Neonatal jaundice. National Institute for Health and Clinical Excellence. 2010. Available at: www.nice.org.uk/CG98. Accessed October 31, 2015.

Index

Note: Page numbers of article titles are in **boldface** type.

Moving?

Make sure your subscription moves with you!

To notify us of your new address, find your **Clinics Account Number** (located on your mailing label above your name), and contact customer service at:

Email: journalscustomerservice-usa@elsevier.com

800-654-2452 (subscribers in the U.S. & Canada)
314-447-8871 (subscribers outside of the U.S. & Canada)

Fax number: 314-447-8029

Elsevier Health Sciences Division
Subscription Customer Service
3251 Riverport Lane
Maryland Heights, MO 63043

*To ensure uninterrupted delivery of your subscription, please notify us at least 4 weeks in advance of move.

Printed and bound by CPI Group (UK) Ltd, Croydon, CR0 4YY

07/10/2024

01040505-0014